Neurosurgery for GP's

Neurosurgery for GP's

W. Adriaan Liebenberg
MMed Neurosurgery (Stellenbosch), FCS Neurosurg (SA)

With contributions from

Lal Gunasekera
Phd, FRCS

VESUVIUS BOOKS LTD
Published by Vesuvius Books Ltd.
Copyright © Vesuvius Books Ltd, 2006

All rights reserved. No part of this publication may be translated into other languages, reproduced, stored in a retrieval system, or transmitted, in any form or by any means, electronic, mechanical, photocopying, recording or otherwise, without prior permission in writing of the publisher.

No responsibility or liability is assumed by either the authors or the publisher for any injury, loss, or damage to persons or property as a matter of products liability, negligence, or otherwise, or from the use or operation of any methods, products, instruments, instructions, or ideas contained in this book. Every effort has been made to ensure that the details given in this book regarding the choice, operation or use of any instrumentation, or the choice, dosage and administration practices relating to pharmaceutical agents, which are mentioned in the text, are in accordance with the recommendations and practices current at the time of publication. However, because new research constantly leads to such recommendations and practices being updated, the reader should obtain independent verification of diagnoses and check the makers' instructions carefully regarding the choice and use of instruments, and regarding the administration practices, doses, indications and contraindications associated with pharmaceutical agents mentioned in this book.

The statements made, and the opinions expressed, in this book are those of the authors and do not necessarily reflect the views of the company or companies which manufacture and/or market any of the instruments or pharmaceutical products referred to, nor do any statement made amounts to an endorsement of the quality or value of such instruments or products, or any claims made by their manufacturers.

ISBN 0-9548813-2-X

Contents

1. Referral to neurosurgery

2. Clinical evaluation

3. Cranial imaging

4. Spinal imaging

5. Headache

6. Brain tumours

7. Degenerative conditions

8. Hydrocephalus

9. Cerebral infarction and haemorrhage

10. Craniospinal infection

11. Vascular abnormalities

1

REFERRAL TO NEUROSURGERY

Contents

Introduction
What information should a referral contain?
Clinical examination
Imaging

Introduction
A patient may be referred to neurosurgery as an elective, urgent or emergency case. As in all surgical specialities, a decision needs to be taken as to whether the management should be conservative or surgical; since many neurosurgical conditions can be managed conservatively, and whether this should be done emergently, urgently or electively. For instance, somebody with a mild lumbar disc herniation may frequently be managed conservatively without surgical intervention, as would a patient who has end-stage, widespread cancer and multiple cranial metastases. On the other hand, for someone who has an intracranial brain abscess or a threatening paralysis from a cauda equina syndrome, surgery is indicated as an emergency. In a prolapsed cervical disc with resultant myelopathy, surgery is indicated on an urgent rather than emergency basis. A patient presenting with an incidental intracranial meningioma without mass effect would also need surgery if the tumour shows progression on follow up imaging but this would be performed as an elective procedure.

A large part of this decision making process happens when the patient is initially referred to neurosurgery and is based on the clinical history and the clinical examination that the referring doctor supplies. It is therefore obvious that as much information as possible is needed in order to make a proper decision which has potentially far reaching consequences for the patient. When taking the history of a patient presenting with a neurological deficit or disease the salient feature is the speed of onset. In cranial pathology, if the speed of onset is fast - within minutes to hours - it is important to ascertain whether this is a transient phenomenon such as a transient ischaemic attack (TIA), or a progressive phenomenon as in somebody with an intracranial mass lesion secondary to a tumour or bleed who rapidly progresses to a coma and death. Transient deficits are the hallmark of underlying pathology that need urgent investigation whereas progressive deficits are the hallmark of underlying pathology which has progressed to the point where it could lead to permanent neurological deficit or death and usually needs emergency investigation and treatment.

Patients who have had long term, ongoing, grumbling symptoms which slowly progress often have an underlying malignancy which has slowly increased in size causing progressive mass effect on the brain. In spinal pathology the speed of onset is also extremely important. Somebody who develops acute, sudden lower back pain with accompanying sciatic pains down their legs will commonly have a ruptured intervertebral disc whereas somebody who is pyrexial, has a focal tenderness in their spine, appears septic and has rapid progressive radicular pains and motor deficit most probably has a compressive extradural empyema collection of the lumbosacral spine. With advancing knowledge of the different types of neurosurgical pathology, the history and clinical examination will in most cases, give you a very accurate differential diagnosis.

What information should a referral contain?
Administrative issues

Name of the referring doctor with grade and speciality.
Who is the responsible senior colleague and what is their contact number.
The name of the patient.
Date of birth and age of the patient.
Is this the patient's normal abode or is the patient out of region (on holiday or business).
Is the patient right- or left-handed (to ascertain hemispheric dominance).
What is the patient's current occupation and, if retired, occupation until retirement.
Which hospital has the patient been referred from.
Which ward is the patient in.

History

Full description of pathology and the temporal course of the disease/event.
Speed of onset (minutes, hours, days, weeks or months).
Is the pathology transient or progressive in nature? Associated symptoms noticed by the patient and also associated symptoms noticed by the family.

Previous medical history.
Important features are markers of vasculopathy like hypertension, angina, myocardial infarction, diabetes mellitus or smoking, previous CVAs and the side of the lesion, epilepsy, previous infections and previous pulmonary pathology. Previous malignancies and status of follow up are also important.

Drug history.
It is very important to ascertain whether the patients are on any blood thinning products, like Aspirin, Warfarin or any other anti-platelet agents and, if they are, what the values of the different clotting parameters are.

Previous level of functioning.

Whether the patient was in full time occupation, was self-caring or needed carers. Whether fully mobile or needed walking aids.

In cases of emergency referrals, at what time did the patient last have a meal and whether the patient is currently nil by mouth.

Clinical examination

The clinical examination will obviously be guided by the history and in cranial patients the emphasis will be different from spinal patients. In cranial patients their level of alertness and the Glasgow Coma Scale is paramount. The Glasgow Coma Scale should be reported as a score out of 15 plus the breakdown. For instance, a patient who localises to pain, mumbles and does not open his eyes should be reported as GCS 8/15 (M5, V2, E1) and a patient who localises to pain, does not open his eyes and is intubated should be reported as GCS 7/15 T (M5, V1, E1(T)). In patients who are mildly to moderately confused the mini mental test score or the abbreviated mini mental test score is a very good way to quantify this.

The next thing of importance in patients with cranial pathology is to establish if there are any focal deficits or long tract signs and the presence or absence of papilloedema (bilateral optic disc swelling) or unilateral optic disc swelling. Patients with severe brain compression due to expansile lesions tend to present with visual inattention or homonymous hemianopias or quadrantopias and hemiparesis involving the arms, leg and face. More subtle abnormalities are, of course, also possible and are dependant on the site of the lesion and the area of the brain that is being compromised.

Patients with intracranial pathology tend to have more generalised deficits than patients with purely spinal disease which obviously occurs lower down in the nervous system where structures have become more specific in their function. When reporting on spinal disease it is important to ascertain any abnormalities of both the motor and the sensory system and for the referring doctors to be very exact in their reporting. Patients who have cervical compressive lesions will either have a radiculopathy (compressing only nerve roots) or myelopathy (compressing the whole of the spinal cord). Patients with radiculopathy will present with pain, paraesthesia and isolated muscle group weakness with a lower motor neurone weakness which means that the reflexes will be depressed. In cases of myelopathy, because the pathology is proximal to the anterior horn cell, patients will present with upper motor neurone weakness which means they will have increased reflexes. Therefore somebody with a central compressive lesion of the spinal cord will be myelopathic and have increased reflexes in their arms and legs with associated weakness. Somebody who has a central compressive lesion in the thoracic spine may have weakness in his legs (paraparesis) and increased reflexes but the function of the muscles and the reflexes of the upper limbs will be normal because they are proximal to the point of pathology. It is therefore of paramount importance to be very exact as to the sensory deficit, motor deficit and reflexes and they should be reported precisely.

As far as the sensory system is concerned, reporting a sensory level will frequently tell us where the lesion is in the spinal cord. For instance a sensory level at T6 usually denotes a spinal cord lesion at T4. The discrepancy between the T4 cord segment and the T6 radicular segment is because the nerve roots do not leave the cord in a perpendicular fashion but angled downwards and leave the outlet foramina at a couple of levels lower down. This is because, during the growth of a human, the bony vertebral column grows more than the spinal cord leading to a dissociation in lengths and therefore the nerve roots actually leave a couple of segments lower down. The pattern of numbness can also tell us about the cord injury as a hemisensory loss is frequently due to a hemi-cord injury (Brown-Séquard syndrome). It is very obvious, therefore, that having a detailed history as well as detailed examination tells us a lot of the type of pathology and allows us to make a diagnosis prior to seeing any imaging. We can then have the luxury of using imaging to confirm our diagnosis. This is especially important with the current new generation of imaging such as the magnetic resonance scan as these are extremely sensitive and can frequently show incidental abnormalities that have no clinical significance.

Imaging

Having provided the neurosurgeon with the clinical history and examination, it is now important for the referring doctor to provide the imaging. This may be either via a digital telelink, or by sending hard copies of the films. It might even be necessary for the neurosurgeon to make a decision based on the report of a radiology colleague within his or her own institution or the referring doctor's own opinion of the scans. If this situation exists it may be useful to look at the chapters on imaging.

2

CLINICAL EVALUATION OF A NEUROSURGICAL PATIENT

Contents

Introduction
History
Physical Examination

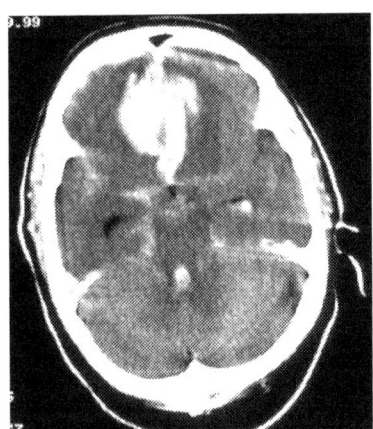

Introduction

Clinical evaluation of a neurosurgical patient as in any other speciality is directed towards arriving at a diagnosis. The diagnosis consists of :

1. Where is the disease? (in terms of anatomy) and
2. What is the disease? (in terms of pathology)

To assist in determining the above you have to take a careful history which will enable you to focus your attention on a particular region of the CNS and conduct a physical examination with emphasis on that particular region. As in other specialties this can involve inspection where the diseased organ can be seen (e.g. the optic fundus), palpation where the organ can be felt (e.g. spinal deformities), and in certain instances auscultation where blood flow changes with disease. These methods have limited direct application to the central nervous system (CNS).

Thus, the diagnosis of a neurological disorder usually requires a different approach. The brain and the spinal cord and even the peripheral nerves are highly specialised structures and in different areas control different functions. Hence if any area in the CNS is diseased, the function controlled by that area will be affected. If you determine what functions are affected in the patient, you can relate these to the area of the CNS involved and thereby determine where the lesion is (in terms of the anatomy). For example, speech is controlled by the speech area situated in the left hemisphere in the temporal region in right handed persons and most left handed persons as well (a proportion of left handed patients have their speech area on the right side). If speech is impaired in a patient, the disease can be localised to the left temporal region of the brain indicating where the lesion is.

The pathology can be determined from the history of onset of the symptoms. The common neurosurgical disorders can be classified as congenital, traumatic, degenerative, inflammatory, neoplastic or vascular diseases. In most congenital disorders the symptoms would be apparent from birth, in traumatic conditions there would be a history of an injury and in inflammatory diseases, there may be features such as pyrexia to suggest infection. As neoplasms grow slowly, the symptoms appear slowly and progress. In vascular diseases blood vessels either get blocked or burst suddenly and the symptoms also are sudden in onset, so much so that the patient or an observer could usually recall exactly what they were doing when it happened. Thus, the history of onset and the progression of symptoms indicate the pathology and the functional impairment determined mainly by the examination points towards the anatomy. Together they help to arrive at the diagnosis.

History

The history is directed mainly towards what functional changes the patient has noticed and the mode of onset and progression. The history should also include a careful past medical history as the present problem may be related to a past illness. The family history is important as many neurological diseases have a hereditary tendency. Drug history and occupational history may indicate exposure to any hazards that could have contributed to the disease. Personal habits such as smoking and alcohol abuse are also relevant in some instances. Social history is important as many neurological diseases can lead to a chronic disability that would have a considerable social impact on the family and friends. Finally a systematic enquiry helps to determine any other co-existing illness which may be relevant to the neurological illness.

Physical Examination

As the diagnosis of neurological diseases involves a careful scrutiny of functional deficits, you have to examine all the functions of the CNS to find out which are impaired. This involves a systematic approach in order not to miss anything and this process constitutes the neurological examination.

The steps involved are:

1. Vital signs
These are pulse rate, blood pressure, respiratory rate and temperature. These signs being measured and expressed in numerical terms are hence objective and any changes can be quantified. They also change with changes of intracranial dynamics and hence form an important aspect in the evaluation and subsequent observation of a neurosurgical patient.

2. Systemic examination
It is preferable for all other systems to be examined first before concentrating on the neurological examination as symptoms of diseases of these systems can mimic neurological diseases (e.g. confusion caused by anoxia). Also, the neurological disturbance could very well be secondary to a systemic illness (e.g. metastatic tumours, cerebral infarcts from cardiac emboli etc.).

3. Neurological examination

Neurological examination
The full and thorough examination of a neurosurgical patient should be a seamless, fast process and comes only with practice. Following the detailed history you will already have a very good idea of what it is that you are dealing with and you can tailor your examination to this. When there is a good understanding of the pathology it becomes quite easy to focus on certain aspects.

Alertness and mental function
Patients with neurological disease frequently have differing levels of consciousness and examination of unconscious patients obviously differs markedly from that of the patient who is conscious, awake and alert. In the patient who is awake the first thing to assess is their mental function and orientation in time, place and person. Two bedside tests are the abbreviated mental test score and the mini mental state examination. See tables 1 and 2.

These are quite rough tools which will not pick up subtle deficiencies, so if these are suspected then assessment by a neuropsychologist is indicated. This is especially true in those patients who are recuperating from an insult to the nervous system such as subarachnoid haemorrhage or traumatic brain injury. It is always good to quantify a baseline in these patients so that progression and improvement can be seen. Following the testing of mental function and orientation of the patient it should be recorded as follows: AMT (score)/10 and MMSE (score)/30 with the orientation noted as "orientated in time, place and person."

Cranial nerves
CN I
The first cranial nerve is frequently involved in tumours of the anterior skull base or in trauma of the anterior skull base and can be tested with different substances. Oil of cloves or coffee is frequently used. The olfactory nerves can be tested independently by pinching the opposite nostril shut and testing one side at a time.

CN II
Visual fields. The second cranial nerve carries visual signals from the retina to the occipital cortex. Compression of the optic nerve or the optic tract and its radiations will lead to deficiencies in the visual field. There will be different clinical manifestations depending on where the compression is. See figure 1. Deficiencies are diagnosed with confrontation testing. See figure 2.

Visual acuity. Visual acuity is tested with a Snellen chart over a set distance of 20 feet and noted as a value which is a fraction of one. Therefore, if the set distance is 20 feet and the patient can see the letters that the chart indicates you should be able to see over a distance of 20 foot and therefore has 20/20 vision, it indicates a value of one, which is normal. If the patient can only see the large letters which you should be able to read at 200 feet then the vision is recorded as 20/200 or 1/10 of normal vision. Countries with the metric system use a Snellen chart that is measured at 6 metres and normal vision is 6/6 vision.

Task	Instructions	Scoring	
Orientation (Date)	"Tell me the date?" Ask for omitted items	One point each for year, season, date, day of week, and month	5
Orientation (Place)	"Where are you?" Ask for omitted items	One point each for state, county, town, building, and floor or room	5
Register 3 objects	Name three objects slowly and clearly. Ask the patient to repeat them	One point for each item correctly repeated	3
Serial sevens	Ask the patient to count backwards from 100 by 7. Stop after five answers. (Or ask them to spell "world" backwards)	One point for each correct answer (or letter)	5
Recall 3 objects	Ask the patient to recall the objects mentioned above	One point for each item correctly remembered	3
Naming	Point to your watch and ask the patient "what is this?" Repeat with a pencil.	One point for each correct answer	2
Repeating a phrase	Ask the patient to say "no ifs, ands, or buts"	One point if successful on first try	1
Verbal commands	Give the patient a plain piece of paper and say "Take this paper in your right hand, fold it in half, and put it on the floor"	One point for each correct action	3
Written commands	Show the patient a piece of paper with "CLOSE YOUR EYES" printed on it	One point if the patient closes their eyes	1
Writing	Ask the patient to write a sentence	One point if sentence has a subject, a verb, and makes sense	1
Drawing	Ask the patient to copy a pair of intersecting pentagons onto a piece of paper	One point if the figure has ten corners and two intersecting lines	1
	A score of 24 or above is considered normal		30

Table 1. *Folstein's Mini Mental Status Examination*

Age	Must be correct
Time	Without looking at watch/clock; correct to nearest hour
42 East Street	Give this address. Check registration. Check memory at end of test.
Month	Exact
Year	Exact, except in Jan/Feb when previous year OK
Name of place	If not in hospital ask type of place or area of town
Date of birth	Exact
Start of WW1	Exact
Name of present monarch/president	Exact
Count backwards from 20 to 1	Can prompt with the first few numbers, but no further prompts, patient can hesitate and self correct but no other errors
Score 8-10	Normal
Score 7	Probably abnormal
Score < 6	Abnormal

Table 2. *Abbreviated Mental Test score. One point for each correct answer.*

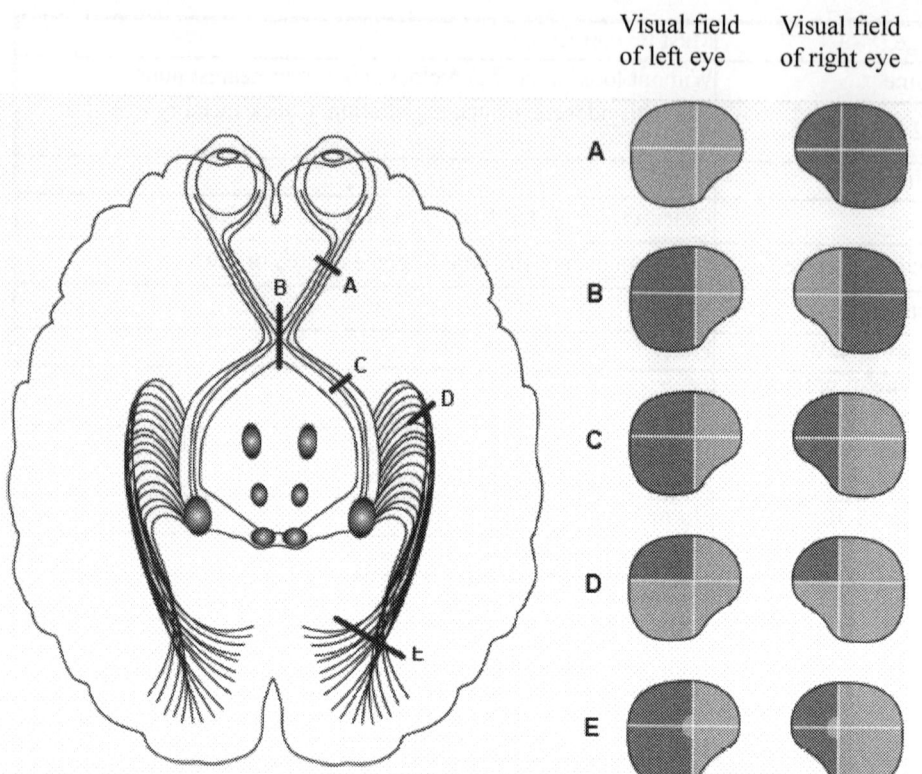

Figure 1. *Visual field deficits according to the site of the compression - A. complete vision loss in right eye, B. bitemporal hemianopia, C. left homonomous hemianopia, D. left upper quadrant hemianopia, E. macular sparing in left homonomous hemianopia. It is important to note that the images transmitted in the nasal fibers of the optic nerve cross over in the chiasm and that the temporal fibers continue straight backwards. It is also important to note that the lower retinal fibers cross anteriorly and the upper retinal fibers cross posteriorly in the chiasm. The lower retinal fibers carry the upper temporal visual field and the upper retinal fibers carry the lower temporal field. Beyond the lateral geniculate body, the fibers fan out into the optic radiation and the fibers serving the lower nasal retina (the upper temporal field) dip into the temporal lobe. These fibers are called Meyer's loop. Compression of these fibers leads to a contralateral upper quadrantanopia. It will be a homonomous hemianopia since the nasal fibers from the contralateral eye would have crossed over in the chiasm. Visual fields can be assessed by visual confrontation testing. See figure 2. The most sensitive way to do this is to use a red pin because red is the first colour that we experience inability to see when there is compression of the optic nerve.*

It is important to remember that patients can have near normal visual acuity with large deficits in their visual fields. Having tested both visual fields and visual acuity it is now important to perform fundoscopy.

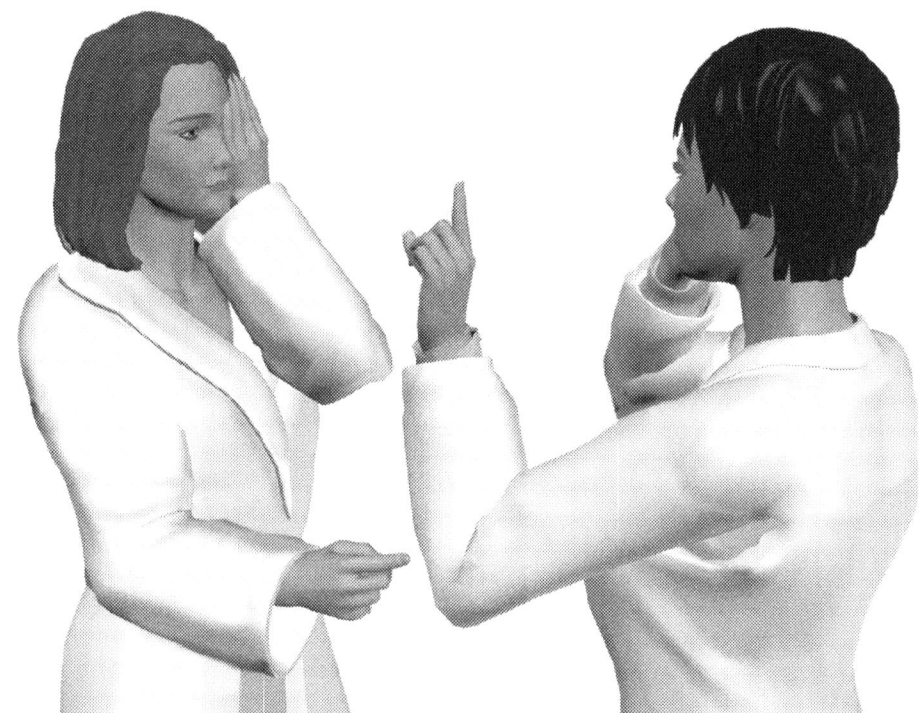

Figure 2. *Visual confrontation testing. Whilst sitting opposite the patient you ask them to occlude their left eye while you occlude your right eye and, using the limits of your own visual field, you test whether the patient has the same extent of visual field. Repeat this with the other eye. Visual fields are recorded as the patient sees them. Therefore the left temporal field will be recorded on the left and the right temporal field on the right.*

Fundoscopy
This is a skill that is learnt only with a lot of practice and it is frequently reported incorrectly. It is important to note that papilloedema (bilateral optic disc swelling) takes 10-14 days to develop and is not present in the patient with acute head injury. It is rather a hallmark of chronic raised intracranial pressure or chronic optic disc pathology. It is frequently said that patients who have no papilloedema are safe to undergo a lumbar puncture without resorting to any cranial imaging. This is incorrect, as a patient who has a large acute subdural haematoma or intracerebral haematoma will not have papilloedema and performing a lumbar puncture on these patients can lead to coning and death.
Papilloedema has four stages. See table 3.

CN III, IV, VI
These three nerves work together to move the eyeball around in its socket. The third cranial nerve has the added function of pupil constriction and carries sympathetic fibres that mediate eyelid elevation. Most of the muscles of the eyeball are supplied by the third cranial nerve, but the *lateral rectus* is supplied by the sixth cranial nerve and the *superior oblique* by the fourth cranial nerve. This causes a patient with a third nerve palsy to have an eyeball which looks downwards and outwards because of the unopposed pull of the *lateral rectus* and *superior oblique muscles*. In cases of *lateral rectus* palsy, the eyeball loses the ability to look laterally. In an isolated fourth nerve palsy, the patient develops diplopia on looking outwards and downwards.

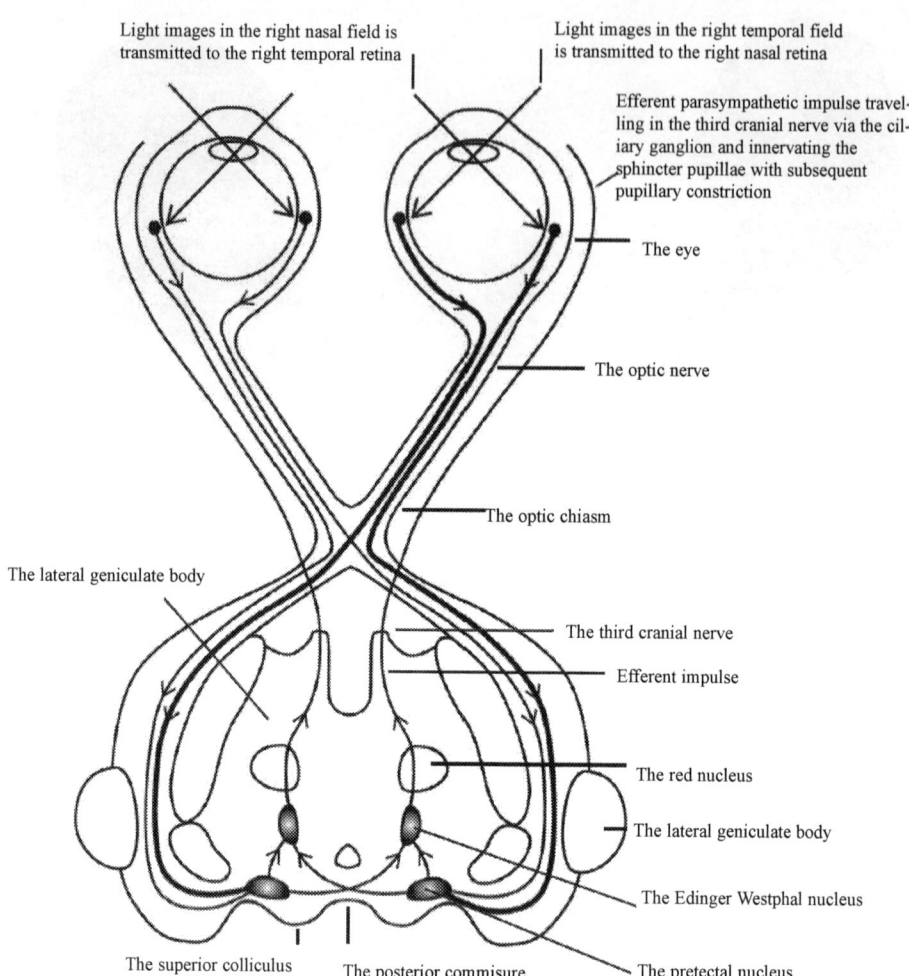

Figure 3. *Pupillary light reflex - pupillary constriction is a parasympathetic function and is mediated by the Edinger Westphal nuclei. Light impulses travel back in the second cranial nerve and in the brain stem at the level of superior colliculus bilaterally innervates the Edinger-Westphal nuclei. Efferent impulses then travel forwards in both third cranial nerves and therefore light shone into one eye activates constriction in both eyes.*

The *superior oblique* pulls the eye downwards and medially as it acts by hooking around the trochlea and the *inferior rectus* pulls the eye down and laterally. In a patient with fourth cranial nerve palsy, downward gaze results in unopposed action of the *inferior rectus* pulling the affected eye downwards and outwards. Downward gaze therefore precipitates or worsens diplopia. Pupillary constriction is a parasympathetic function and is mediated by the Edinger-Westphal nuclei. Light impulses travel back in the second cranial nerve and in the brain stem at the level of superior colliculus bilaterally innervates the Edinger Westphal nuclei. Efferent impulses then travel forwards in both third cranial nerves and therefore light shone into one eye activates constriction in both eyes, see figure 3.

Stage one	There is decreased drainage of the veins of the optic nerve and this leads to the veins swelling and becoming tortuous. An experienced observer will also be able to see decreased venous pulsation
Stage two	The optic discs swell and, where the vessels of the optic disc in the normal situation have an acute posterior kink plunging into the optic discs, they now stop at the margin of the disc. The discs frequently changes colour from a pale yellow to pink as this occurs
Stage three	The disc margins swell more and become increasingly indistinct and blurred
Stage four	There is even more swelling of the discs with obvious elevation and scattered haemorrhages frequently seen

Table 3. *Grades of papilloedema*

If there is compression or dysfunction of the afferent pathway of the pupillary reflex (second cranial nerve) this will lead to a Marcus Gunn pupil: light falling on the affected pupil will lead to a larger pupil than when light falls on the unaffected pupil. This is due to the ipsilateral input to the Edinger Westphal nucleus being weaker (because of the damage to the afferent pathway) than when light is shone into the contralateral eye with the unaffected optic nerve (consensual light reflex). This is demonstrated by swinging a flashlight between the two eyes and seeing a slight dilatation when the light falls directly on the affected eye. Compression of the efferent pathway (third cranial nerve), causes dysfunction of pupil constriction and that leads to a persistently dilated pupil. The pupillary constrictor fibres lie quite superficially in the third nerve and a hallmark of external compression is that of pupillary dilatation. The third nerve also carries sympathetic fibres which innervate the superior tarsal muscles and assist eye opening. Thus a patient with an external compressive third nerve lesion will have a dilated pupil, ptosis and a downward and outward deviated eye (ophthalmoplegia). Pupillary dilatation is a sympathetic activity and is initiated in the hypothalamus with the signals descending in the spinal cord to the level of T1. At the level of T1, the white rami of the nerve roots of C8 and T1 pass through the cervical sympathetic ganglion. Impulses travel from there in sympathetic nerves into the cranial cavity on the surface of the carotid artery and arrive at the pupil via a branch of the ophthalmic artery. When there is dysfunction of the sympathetic system it leads to ptosis because of the decreased innervation of the tarsal muscles, pupillary constriction due to a loss of pupillary dilatation and loss of facial sweating due to autonomic dysfunction. This is called Horner's syndrome and is easily remembered by the rhyme "ptosis, myosis and anhydrosis." The pupillary abnormality is best demonstrated by taking the patient into a darkened room. In normal circumstances, both pupils will dilate in a darkened room but in a patient with Horner's syndrome, the affected pupil will remain constricted.

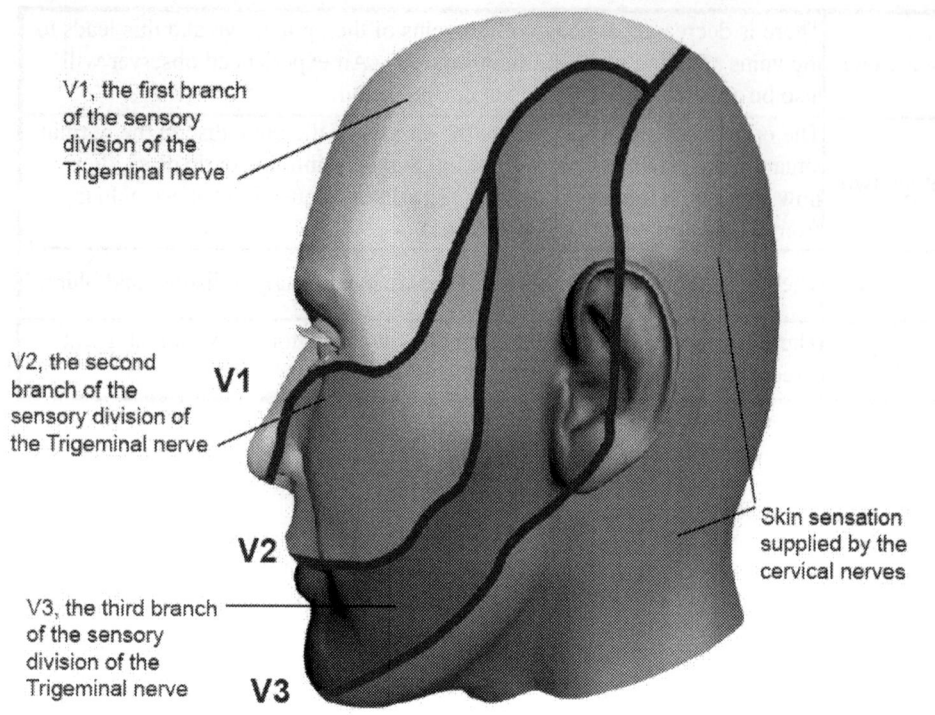

Figure 4. *Distribution of the Trigeminal nerve's sensory divisions. Note that the sensation in front of the tragus is supplied by the 7th and 9th cranial nerves (not demonstrated)*

CN V
The first division of the fifth cranial nerve accompanies the third, fourth and sixth cranial nerves through the cavernous sinus and these four nerves are frequently compromised together by lesions in the cavernous sinus. The fifth cranial nerve's largest component is the sensory division but it also has a motor division that serves mastication. It is assessed by testing sensation over the face and by testing corneal sensation (first division) and the jaw jerk. It is important to realise that the first division of the fifth cranial nerve actually supplies sensation as far back as the coronal suture, but does not supply the jaw line. See figure 4.

CN VII
The seventh cranial nerve is almost purely made up of motor fibers and supplies the muscles of the face. The facial nerve has a supranuclear input which supplies the ipsilateral side of the face and also a reflex component that is primarily concerned with reflex eye closure and has no cortical component. Both eyes will shut if there is danger to either individual eye and therefore there is dual innervation of both sides of the forehead. If there is dysfunction of the cortical innervation (supranuclear innervation) this leads to deficient lower face muscle function and intact upper face function. The seventh cranial nerve also has a small sensory function and carries sensation from the external auditory canal and taste sensation from the anterior two-thirds of the tongue via the chorda tympani.

CN VIII
The vestibulocochlear nerve consists of the vestibular nerve and the cochlear nerve. The

vestibular nerve serves balance and the cochlear nerve hearing. Hearing can be tested by rubbing your fingers next to the patient's ears and determining whether they can hear that or, alternatively, whispering numbers in their ears and asking the patient to relay which numbers have been whispered. Weber and Rinne's tests are useful in distinguishing between conductive and sensory neural deafness. Weber's test consists of placing a vibrating tuning fork on the patient's vertex and asking if the patient feels or hears it best on one side or the other. A patient with no abnormalities will experience no difference. In cases with unilateral neurosensory hearing loss, the hearing will be best in the normal ear, while in cases of a unilateral conductive hearing loss, it is best heard in the abnormal ear. In Rinne's test, bone conduction (placing the tuning fork on the mastoid process) is compared to air conduction (placing the tuning fork in front of but not touching the pinna). Normally, air conduction is greater than bone conduction. In cases of partial neurosensory hearing loss, air conduction is still greater than bone conduction but in cases of conduction hearing loss bone conduction will be greater than air conduction. It is sometimes difficult to remember which test does what but I remember Weber's test as being the one where you put the tuning fork on top of somebody's head by the fact that a 'W' looks a bit like a crown.

CN IX, X, XI

These nerves share the same motor nucleus (nucleus ambiguus) and all exit the skull through the jugular foramen. The **glossopharyngeal nerve (IX)** is the main afferent pathway of the gag reflex and also, along with the seventh cranial nerve, supplies some sensation in the external auditory canal and conveys taste, in this case, from the posterior third of the tongue. The only function that we routinely test is the gag reflex and the efferent pathway of the gag reflex is the tenth cranial nerve **(vagus)**. The tenth cranial nerve also supplies motor fibres to the muscles of the palate. Testing the ninth and tenth nerves together then consists of testing the gag reflex and also testing the patient's palatal muscles by asking them to open their mouth widely and saying "aaaahh" whilst using a light to illuminate the back of the mouth. If there is a palsy of the vagus, there will be asymmetry of the palate and a left-sided nerve palsy will cause the intact muscles on the right-hand side to pull the palate over to the right and vice-versa. Having a depressed gag reflex can either be because of dysfunction in the ninth or tenth cranial nerve. Patients with a ninth nerve palsy will usually have normal palatal function. The gag is tested by stimulating the uvula and posterior pharynx with a tongue depressor. The tenth cranial nerve also supplies the larynx and a vagal or recurrent laryngeal nerve palsy causes ipsilateral vocal cord paralysis and a hoarse voice.

The **spinal accessory nerve (XI)** originates in a nucleus in the spinal cord and leaves the spinal cord through the cervical branches supplying the *sternocleidomastoid and trapezius muscles* on the same side. The unusual feature of this nerve is that the higher control is not crossed and a right-sided lesion will therefore lead to a right-sided nerve dysfunction. The *sternocleidomastoid muscle* pulls the patient's head towards the opposite side and right *sternocleidomastoid muscle* (right eleventh nerve) function is therefore tested by asking the patient to look towards the left against resistance and simultaneously palpating the muscles on the right-hand side. A patient with a right hemisphere lesion will not be able to look towards the left-hand side and if we remember the anatomy of the second cranial nerve, they will have inattention of the left visual field. Therefore patients with extensive right hemisphere damage will not be aware of the left-hand side and will not be able to look towards the left-hand side.

CN XII

The twelfth cranial nerve supplies the motor function of the tongue and is tested by both observation and active movement. Observing the tongue lying in the floor of the mouth with the patient's mouth open will demonstrate any fasciculation if present. The patient is then asked to push the tongue out of their mouth and move it from side to side. If there is a palsy, the stronger intact muscles will push the tongue towards the affected weaker side and there

CN I	Usually reserved for cases where the patient reports a decrease in olfaction
CN II	Visual confrontation, acuity and fundoscopy
CN III, IV, VI	Eye movements
CN V	Facial sensation
CN VII	Facial movements
CN VIII	Rubbing your fingers next to the ear (Rinne, Weber)
CN IX - XII	Gag reflex, palatal function, shoulder and neck movements and looking at tongue movements

Table 4. *Examination of the cranial nerves*

fore the tongue will deviate towards the affected side (whereas in the case of a tenth nerve palsy, the palate will pull away from the affected side). This can be remembered by the fact that the tongue muscles push out and the palatal muscles pull up. See table 4 for a summary of the cranial nerve examination.

Examination of the motor system

The left hemisphere controls the right-hand side of the body and vice versa. The motor system is made up of two parts: the main controlling pyramidal system (named after the pyramids in the medulla oblongata) and the extrapyramidal system which modulates the pyramidal system and does not cross over. Motor signals are generated in the cortex and then travel via the corona radiata and the internal capsule down to the brainstem. They cross over in the medulla oblongata to the opposite side to control motor movement. The extrapyramidal system modulates the actions of the pyramidal system based on proprioception and feedback via the cerebellum. In a hemispheric deficit there is dysfunction of the motor system on the whole of the contralateral side. A large left hemispheric infarct will produce a paralysis of the right side of the face, the right arm and the right leg. Because the reflex arc of the spinal cord is independent of cerebral input, patients who are completely paralysed will still have intact reflexes. Reflexes are however modulated by higher input and if there is dysfunction anywhere in the brain or the spinal cord the effect downstream of that will be a decrease in modulation of the reflex activity. Therefore patients who have a left hemisphere infarct will have spastic right arm and leg reflexes due to non-modulated reflex arc activity. This is also true if the cause of the paralysis is in the spinal cord which will lead to decreased muscle power below the level of the lesion and increase in the reflexes (hyperreflexia). This is extremely useful in delineating the level of the pathology. Somebody who has damage to the spinal cord at C6 level will have increased reflexes below the level of C6 as well as weakness below that level with normal power and reflexes above that level. The rule for establishing the level of spinal pathology is that at the level of injury there will be decreased reflexes and weakness (lower motor neurone signs) and below the level there will be weakness and increased reflexes (upper motor neurone signs). Lesions distal to the anterior horn cells in the spinal cord lead to lower motor neurone signs (decreased or absent reflexes and weakness). Patients who have only dysfunction of a nerve root might have a radiculopathy and the myotome as well as the dermatome served by this nerve will show dysfunction. For instance somebody with a centrally herniated intervertebral disc (slipped disc) at the L4/5 lumbar level might have a L5 radiculopathy which, if it only involves the sensory component will produce numbness on the dorsum of the foot. If it is severe and also involves the motor component, they will have difficulty with extension (dorsiflexion) of their ankle. When examining the motor system you have to test the tone of the muscles, the muscle power (table 6) and reflexes (table 5).

Description	Score
Absent	-4
Just elicitable	-3
Low	-2
Moderately low	-1
Normal	0
Brisk	1
Very brisk	2
Exhaustible clonus	3
Continuous clonus	4

Table 5. *Mayo Clinic scale for tendon reflex assessment*

Score	Muscle Response
0	No Movement
1	Muscle belly moves but the joint does not move
2	Joint moves with gravity eliminated
3	Joint moves against gravity
4	Joint moves against gravity and some resistance
5	Full strength

Table 6. *MRC Scale for Grading Muscle Strength*

Extrapyramidal system (cerebellar function)
Pathology in the cerebellum causes ipsilateral deficits so that an infarct of the left cerebellum will lead to left-sided weakness and hypotonia. It is important to note that extrapyramidal weakness is not associated with hyperreflexia. Pathology causes a dysfunctional proprioception feedback system and will cause the limbs on the ipsilateral side to be ataxic. Lesions of the vermis, on the other hand, will lead to truncal ataxia. Limb ataxia can be tested by checking the patient for past pointing with the ability to do the finger-nose test and testing for the presence of dysdiadocokinesia. In the lower limbs ataxia can be tested by asking the patient to tap his foot on the floor or to do the heel-to-shin test. Another marker of possible cerebellar pathology is nystagmus.

Muscles	Root Levels	Clinical
Trapezius	C3-C4	Shrug shoulders
Deltoid	C5-C6	Abduct shoulder
Biceps	C5-C6	Flex elbow
Triceps	C6-C8	Extend elbow
Wrist extensors	C6-C7	Extend wrist
Wrist flexors	C6-T1	Flex wrist
Hand intrinsic muscles	C8-T1	Spread fingers
Opponens pollicis and digiti minimi	C8-T1	Make "o" with thumb and 5th finger
Iliopsoas	L2-L3	Flex hip
Quadriceps	L3-L4	Extend knee
Hamstrings	L5-S1	Flex knee
Gluteus maximus	S1-S2	Extend hip
Tibialis anterior	L4-L5	Dorsiflex foot
Tibialis posterior	L4-5	Invert foot
Peroneii	L5-S1	Evert foot
Extensor hallucis longus	L5	Extend (dorsiflex) great toe
Gastrocnemius	S1-S2	Plantar flexion

Table 7. *Myotomes*

Tendon	Root
Bicep reflex	C5/6
Brachioradialis reflex	C6
Triceps	C7
Patella (knee) reflex	L4
Achilles (ankle) reflex	S1

Table 8. *Deep tendon reflexes*

Gait

The last part of evaluation of the motor system is to test the patient's gait. A lot can be learned from a patient's gait. Patients with severe lower back pain and radicular pain will have a type of gait where they put less pressure on the affected side and walk with a limp. This is called an antalgic type of gait. Patients who have suffered cerebrovascular accidents, often have a fixed flexion of their upper limb and a straight, outstretched leg with a plantar-flexed foot which causes them to walk by circumducting the affected leg. They do this by swinging the stiff leg out and around before putting it down. Where there is cerebellar pathology the patient may have a general unsteadiness due to limb ataxia. Patients who are myelopathic have a stiff, spastic gait and frequently shuffle along.

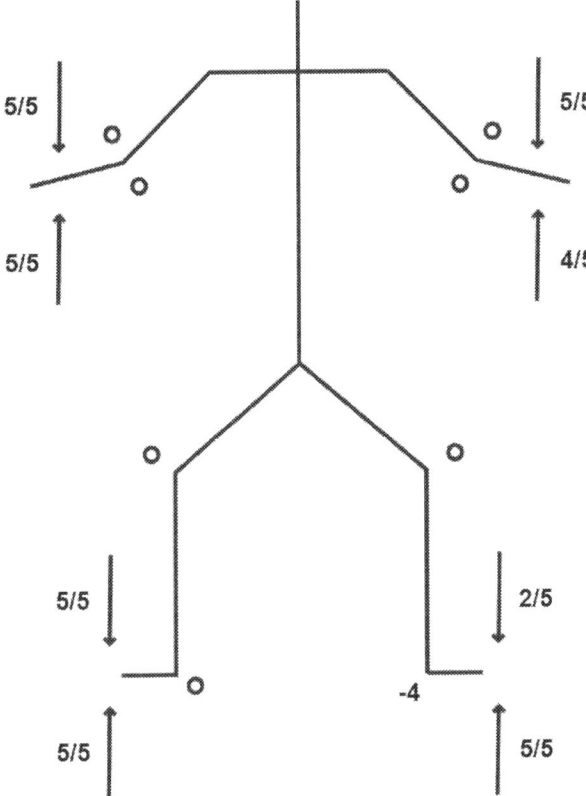

Figure 6. *Notation of the motor system examination. The motor strength (Table 6) and reflexes (Table 5) should be noted on a visual chart as above.*

Romberg
Following assessment of gait you may want to do a Romberg's test. Romberg's test is based on the fact that we need at least 2 out of 3 senses to be able to stand unaided (proprioception, vestibular function, vision). If patients close their eyes and they have a deficit in either their vestibular function or proprioception, they will fall over. This is, however, not a very specific test.

Overview of the motor examination
The suggested sequence for examining the motor system is as follows:
Ask the patient to hold their arms stretched out in front of them with palms upward facing. Ask them to close their eyes. Any subtle weakness will result in a drift of the arm on the weak side. Now ask the patient to open their eyes, turn their palms downwards towards the floor and to make piano playing movements with their fingers. If they can do this, you have successfully screened for subtle motor weakness. You have also tested proprioception and fine motor movements and therefore have tested both pyramidal and extrapyramidal systems. This can be followed up by testing tone in all 4 limbs, one at a time and then testing motor function in all the myotomes. The last step is to test the reflexes. Examination for the motor system should be noted down as demonstrated in figure 6.

Examination of the sensory system
When testing the sensory system it is always very important to ask the patient whether they are aware of any abnormal sensation. If they are not then it is unlikely that you will find any deficit. In testing for sensation it is important to test the different sensory modalities (light touch, temperature, pain and joint position sense).

If you are testing for pain it usually negates the necessity to test for temperature sensation as well, except in patients where we have reason to suspect hydromyelia or syringomyelia where the loss of temperature sensation is quite typical. We therefore effectively have 3 modalities that we test for – proprioception, the fibres of which are located in the posterior part of the spinal cord, light touch, the fibres of which are located in the anterior part of the spinal cord and pain, the fibres of which are located in the lateral part of the spinal cord. Light touch can be tested by running your fingertips or cotton wool lightly along the patient's skin. Pain sensation is tested with a pinprick. Proprioception and joint position sense is tested by moving the patient's toes, feet, fingers or hands with their eyes closed. When testing pain sensation it is important to realise that the pain fibres cross over in the spinal cord and not at the brain stem unlike the other fibres. Therefore a lesion that is restricted to only one half of the spinal cord will lead to ipsilateral proprioceptive and light touch abnormalities, and contralateral pain sensation abnormalities below the affected spinal level (dermatome). This is the basis for the Brown-Séquard syndrome.

It is important not to fall in the C4/T2 trap and to realise that the dermatomes on the chest for C4 and T2 are close to each other and therefore a C4 lesion can be mistaken for a thoracic lesion if the sensation in the arms is not tested. Somebody who is numb from just above the level of their nipples downwards and therefore has a sensory level just above their nipples might have a T3/4 lesion but, if you were to examine their arms that contain the cervical dermatomes and find that they were numb as well, you would have to conclude that this was actually a cervical rather than a thoracic lesion. See figure 7 for the anatomical pattern of dermatomes. Another type of sensory deficit is a cortical sensory deficit and patients with lesions in their parietal lobe might have a deficiency in two point discrimination and discrimination of objects.

Examination of the comatose patient
Examination of the comatose patient is restricted to testing the pupillary reactivity, the Glasgow Coma Scale, the presence of a paresis or paralysis and the patient's reflexes including pathological reflexes (Babinski). The Glasgow Coma Scale is made up of the motor response, the verbal response and eye opening.

The motor response comprises 6 points. See table 8. The notation for a patient's GCS is as follows: GCS (total score)/15, M (score), V (score), E (score). Patients who are intubated have an annotated T added to indicate intubation (GCS 7/15 T). Following notation of the GCS, the pupillary activity is then noted and the term "PEARL" can be used which stands for pupils equal and reactive to light. Following notation of the GCS and the pupillary activity, the focal deficit must be noted down for paresis or paralysis of any of the limbs. Verbal response is scored out of 5. It needs to be remembered that someone who has a lesion focally in Broca's area will not be able to speak properly and will therefore drop several points on the Glasgow Coma Scale. Therefore somebody with a Glasgow Coma Scale of 11/15 may be completely awake and orientated, but completely aphasic, see table 9 for a summary of the verbal response. Eye opening response is scored out of 4. See table 10 for a summary of the eye opening response.

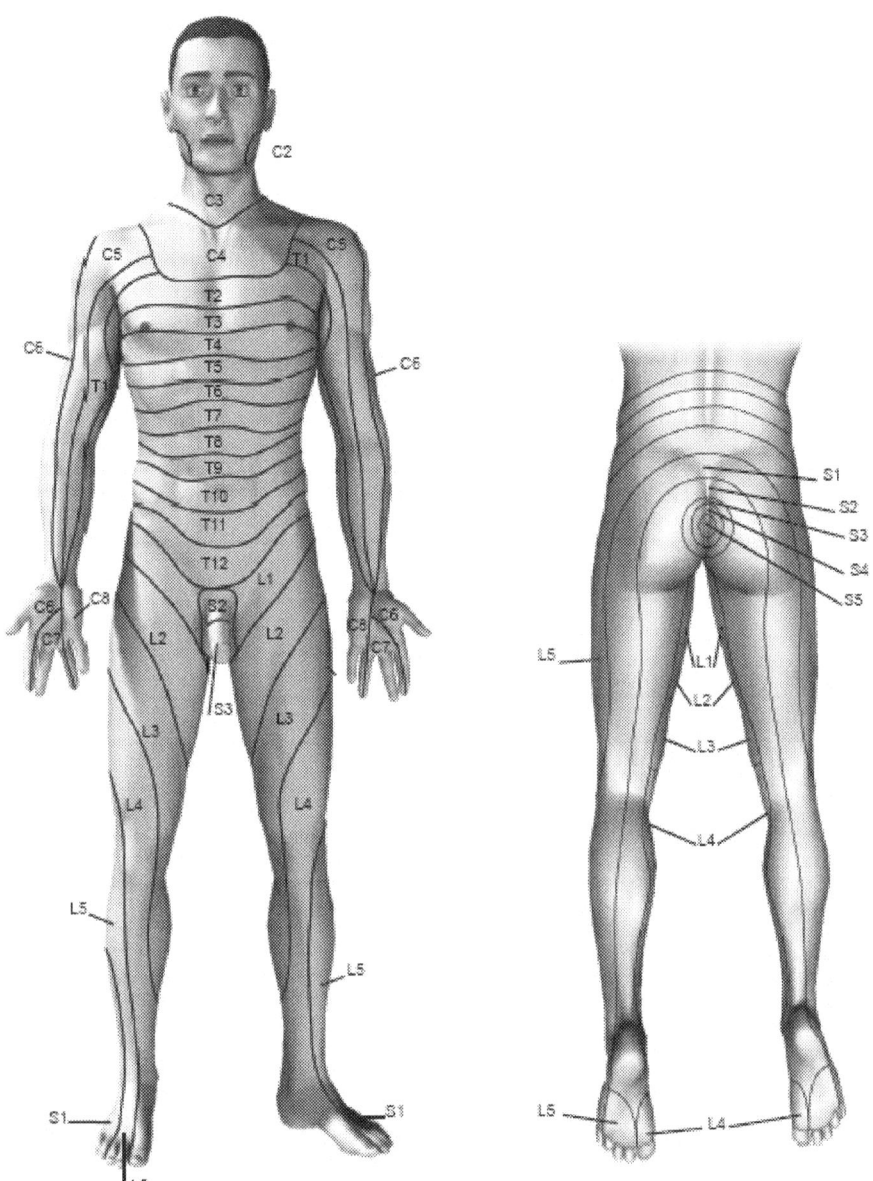

Figure 7. *Human dermatomes*

6/6	Ability to follow commands which requires a rather sophisticated train of events to occur in the nervous system
5/6	The awareness and localisation of painful stimuli. Painful stimulus on the chest wall will therefore lead to the patient grasping your hand and even trying to pull it away
4/6	The patient is aware of the pain or threat and attempts to localise it but cannot. Patients who flex their limbs but are unable to localise the painful stimulus.
3/6	The patient's arms are spasmodically fully flexed next to the body. This is an action that has no reliance on cognition of the cortex and is therefore called decorticate posturing
2/6	The arms are spasmodically extended on either side of the body; the legs are also spastic and extended. This is a final reflex stage that does not rely on the cerebrum at all and so it is called decerebrate posturing. Posturing, both decorticate and decerebrate carry a poor prognosis
1/6	No motor response. Therefore somebody who has even a flicker of movement will get a score of 2/6

Table 8. *Motor response (GCS)*

5/5	Patient is fully orientated to person, time and place
4/5	Confused speech
3/5	Words only
2/5	Sounds only
1/5	No sound whatsoever

Table 9. *Verbal response (GCS)*

4/4	The patient spontaneously opens the eyes
3/4	The patient opens the eyes to verbal stimuli
2/4	The patient opens the eyes to painful stimuli
1/4	The patient does not open the eyes at all

Table 10. *Eye opening response*

3

CRANIAL IMAGING

Contents

CT scans
MRI scans
An approach to reading scans and radiological anatomy
Hydrocephalus and ventriculomegaly
Trauma
Brain tumours

CT scans

A Computed Tomography scan is a process where ordinary X-rays (tomograms) are fed through a computer (computed - therefore the term computed tomography) to form a 2D or 3D picture. Different tissues have different densities to X-ray penetration and are reported as hypo, iso and hyperdense. Iodine based contrast is used to enhance areas of increased blood flow or capillary leakage which show up as more dense areas on CT scans since these areas have a higher load of radiodense contrast material.

Tissue densities:
There are four shades of grayscale that tissues can have on a CT scan: white, grey, dark grey and black.
White (hyperdense)
Bone
Calcium deposits
Blood (fresh)
Melanin
Contrast enhancement
Grey (isodense)
Brain
Glial tumours
Blood (subacute)
Dark grey (hypodense)
Most fluid is seen as dark grey, quite close to pure black and if there are different densities, it usually indicates deposits within the fluid.
CSF (ventricles, subarachnoid spaces)
Brain oedema
Fat
Dermoid tumours are black due to fatty deposits
Blood (chronic)
Black (hypodense)
Air

Hounsfield units
The pixels that make up a CT scan image are assigned a numerical value and these values can be used to identify the type of tissue shown on the image. These values range between -1000 for air and +1000 for bone and water is designated as 0. Fat generally has a value of -50 and soft tissues a value of +40.

MRI scans
Physics
Magnetic Resonance Imaging is a process where the body's hydrogen atoms are aligned by a strong magnet (the magnetic part) and is then subjected to powerful radio wave frequencies that are used to push them out of alignment. The hydrogen atoms alternately absorb and emit radio wave energy, vibrating backwards and forwards between their magnetised resting state and their agitated state caused by the radio pulses (the "resonance" part of MRI). Depending on how quickly these atoms return to their original state, the computer can deduce what kind of tissue is represented by the signals returned. This is based on the intensities of the returned signal and therefore the tissues are reported as being hypo, iso and hyperintense (compared to *densities* in CT scans). A paramagnetic contrast medium, Gadolinium is used in a similar fashion as iodine-based contrast is used in CT scans.

Sequences
The different imaging techniques generated by the radio frequency pulses are called pulse sequences. They include amongst other, spin-echo, inversion recovery, gradient echo and FLAIR (fluid attenuation inversion recovery) sequences. By changing the scan repetition time (TR - the time between RF pulses) and the echo time (TE - the time between the RF pulse and recording the MR signal), it is possible to change the sequence. The two main types of MRI sequences that are used are T1 and T2 weighted images. The terms T1 and T2 refer to the relaxation of the excited nuclei to their original alignment after being excited by the radio waves (relaxation times).

A variant T1-weighted image (T1 WI) is the **STIR** (short tau inversion recovery) sequence which removes bright fat that obscures the signal of interest in orbital or spine images, with pathology being conspicuously bright.
Proton density is neither a T1 nor a T2-weighted image (T2 WI) and is designed to minimise the effects of T1 and T2 WI. Proton density is the concentration of protons in the tissue in the form of water and macromolecules.
FLAIR (fluid attenuation inversion recovery) sequences are a variant of T2 WI where normal body water is suppressed to show pathological oedematous tissue, which is conspicuously bright.
T1 WI are useful in delineating anatomy and return high intensity signals in the following tissues:
Fat
Melanin
Subacute blood
Fluids with high protein content
Paramagnetic contrast agents

T2 WI are very sensitive to most types of pathology and tissues that return high intensity signals are:
Fluid collections (CSF, tissue oedema)
Infarcted brain
Demyelination
Infection
Neoplasms (most)

T1 WI and T2 WI
Flowing blood moves through the plane of the imaging and does not remain present long enough for the spinning hydrogen atoms to return their signal and therefore return little or no signal. Flowing blood is therefore dark on both T1 WI and T2 WI and the signal returned is referred to as a flow void. Air, calcification (bone) and fibrous tissue also return little or no signal due to a paucity of mobile protons and appear dark on both sequences.

Tissue intensities
White matter, because of its high lipid and low water content, is hypointense (relative to grey matter) on T2 WI and hyperintense on T1 WI. On the other hand, grey matter has higher water content than white matter and will therefore be less intense on T1 WI and more intense on T2 WI. CSF therefore appears dark on T1 WI and has a very high signal on T2 WI. The pituitary gland and infundibulum appear grey on T1 WI and T2 WI. When disease processes infiltrate the white matter and displace the hydrophobic tissue with more hydrophilic tissue, the intensities decrease on T1 WI and increase on T2 WI. Most brain tumours return decreased signal intensity on T1 WI and increased signal intensity on T2 WI. In general, pathological processes increase the water content of tissues and appear bright on T2 WI and have decreased signal on T1 WI but there are a few important exceptions to this rule:
Blood (subacute) and melanin is intrinsically bright (white) on T1 WI.
Tumours with a high nuclear to cytoplasmic ration such as lymphomas and primitive neuroectodermal tumours (PNET) are also iso/ hyperintense on T1 WI.
Multiple areas of increased signal intensity on T2 WI raise the suspicion of secondary metastatic disease, demyelination or vascular disease.

Blood changes with time on MR scans
Depends on age of clot
In T1 WI – remember '**B**ig **G**reat **W**hite **B**ear!'
Hyperacute, within hours - **B**lack (hypointense)
Acute stage, less than 3 days - **G**rey (isointense),
Subacute stage, 3 to 14 days - **W**hite (hyperintense),
Chronic stage, more than 14 days - **B**lack (hypointense)

In T2 WI – remember '**B**ear, **W**hat **B**ear?'
Acute stage – **B**lack (hypointense)
Subacute – **W**hite (hyperintense)
Subacute stage and chronic stages – **B**lack (hypointense)

An approach to reading scans and radiological anatomy
Both MRI and CT scan images are presented as slices through different parts of the skull and brain. On the scan there is usually a scout or survey image that shows a lateral view of the head and neck with lines that have corresponding numbers on them. This is a road map to the slices that can be seen in the rest of the scan. Following the road map indicates which of the axial slices go where in the 3-dimensional anatomic model, see figure 1. About a quarter of the way down through the cranium the ventricles start to appear. They can be discerned from the brain, which is grey, by the fact that they are darker in colour, and nearly pitch black on CT scans and T1 WI and hyperintense on T2 WI. The ventricular system consists of a pair of lateral ventricles, the third ventricle and a fourth ventricle. The third and fourth ventricles are connected by the aqueduct of Sylvius, which we can see on a MRI scan, but not a CT scan. The lateral ventricles have frontal and occipital horns and, in cases of hydrocephalus, we can see the temporal horns of the lateral ventricles. The third ventricle is usually slit-like but in

cases of hydrocephalus and obstruction will become round and distended. The fourth ventricle is in the posterior fossa below the level of the tentorium cerebelli and is usually sickle-shaped. The bone of the cranium is brilliant white on CT scans. Just like ordinary X-rays, the tissues that are relatively impenetrable to the rays are recorded as white on the final film and tissues that allow the rays to pass through are darker in colour.

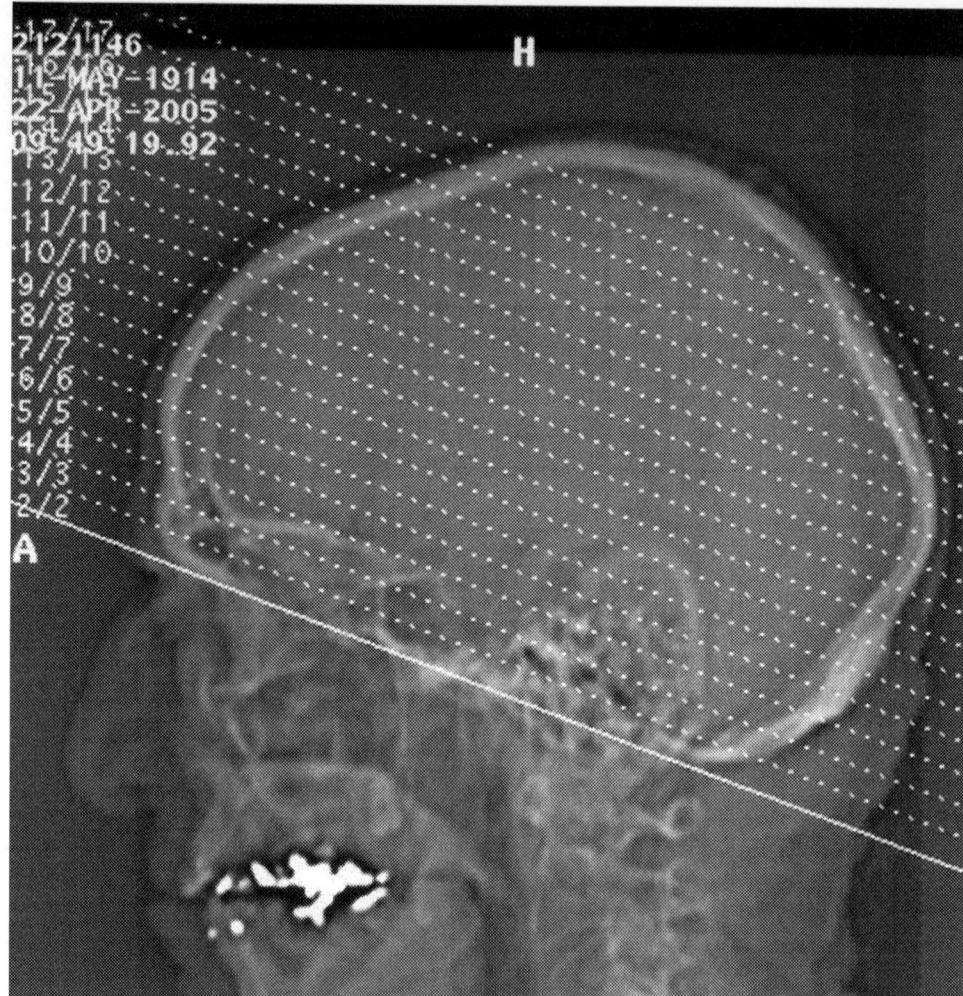

Figure 1. *Note how the CT scan contains a topogram or scout view in the top left hand corner which is a lateral view of the skull with lines running through it. These lines have numbers and the slices that follow are axial images and have corresponding numbers on them so that we can identify through which part of the cranium they were taken. On the opposite page, the bottom slices are small and have a lot of bone and very little brain in them as they are in the uppermost part of the cranium and as we travel through the brain, and move up the scan, the slices become progressively larger.*

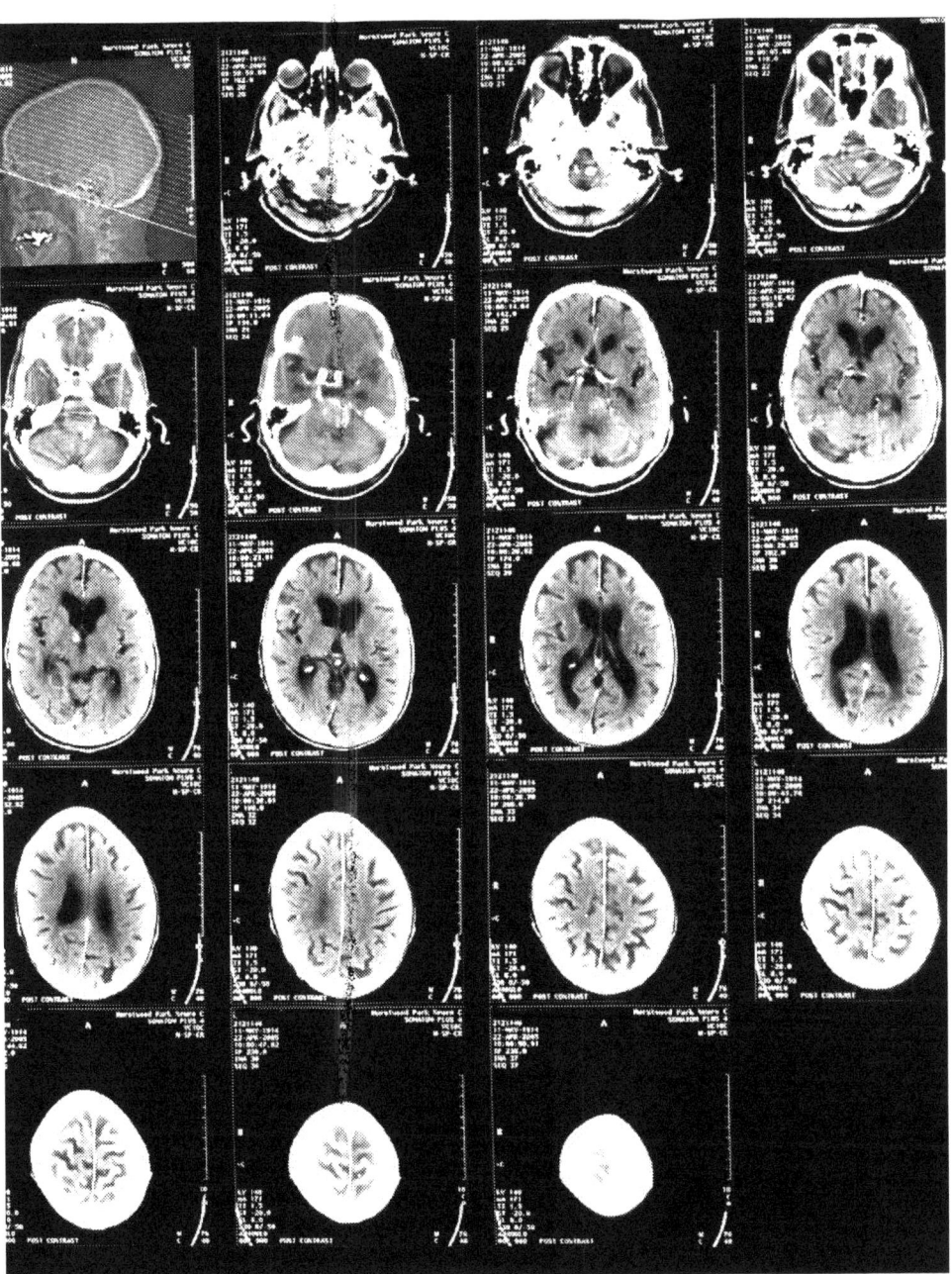

Figure 2. Note how the size of the images changes as the cuts move from top to bottom through the cranial space. In this electronic image, the uppermost images correspond to the top of the cranium as opposed to the other way around on the hard copy seen in figure 1. Note the lateral ventricles as denoted by the white arrow and the white of the calcified choroid plexus in the trigone of the right lateral ventricle as denoted by the black arrow

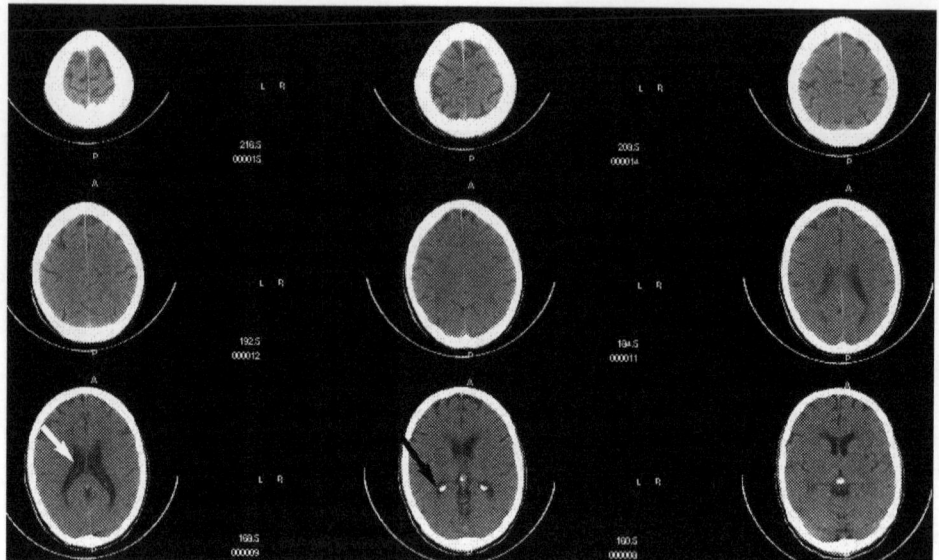

Figure 3. Note the falx (top white arrow), denoting the supratentorial space and how on the next slice, the falx disappears and the top of the posterior fossa is demonstrated (top black arrow). Note the basal cisterns as demonstrated by the bottom white arrow and the brainstem as denoted by the bottom black arrow. The basal cisterns have a fluid density as they contain CSF.

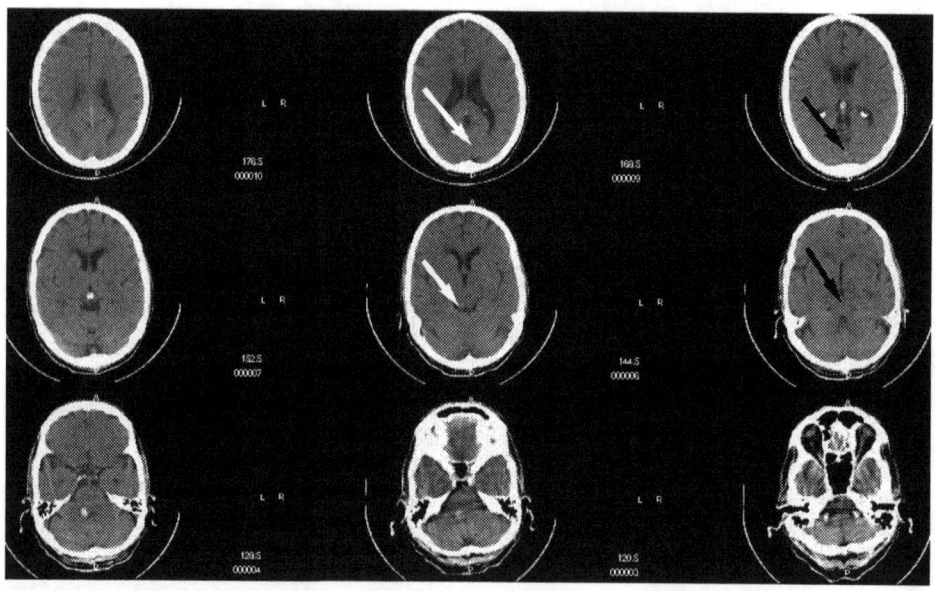

Bone is dark on MRI (T1 WI and T2 WI) because of the calcium deposited in it. At the edges of the brain adjacent to the bone, there are fluid-filled spaces, the subarachnoid spaces, and these are the same colour as the ventricles (dark on CT scan and T1 WI and white on T2 WI) since both contain CSF.

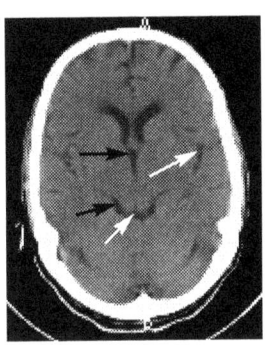

Figure 4. *This is an uncontrasted axial CT scan. The top black arrow indicates the slit like third ventricle, the bottom black arrow the ambient cistern, the bottom white arrow the quadrigeminal cistern and the top white arrow the sylvian fissure.*

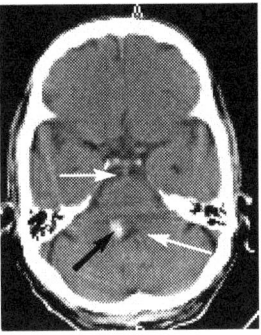

Figure 5. *This is an uncontrasted axial CT scan. The top arrows shows the pre pontine cistern and the bottom arrow the fourth ventricle, which in this case contains fresh blood (black arrow).*

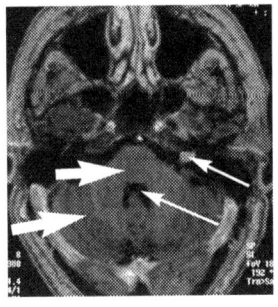

Figure 6. *This is a contrast enhanced axial T1 WI. The top thick arrow demonstrates the pons and the bottom thick arrow demonstrates the cerebellum. The top thin arrow demonstrates a small intracanalicular vestibular schwannoma in the cerebellopontine angle and the bottom thin arrow demonstrates the sickle shaped fourth ventricle.*

Just posterior to the third ventricle, the brain stem can be seen with the basal cisterns around it. These consist of the prepontine, ambient and quadrigeminal cisterns. The supratentorial space is separated from the infratentorial space by the tentorium cerebelli. In the supratentorial space you will see the two cerebral hemispheres seperated by the falx cerebrum. Immediately below the level of the tentorium, the falx is no longer visible and this is the anatomical space of the posterior fossa in which the cerebellum is housed. The cerebellum abuts the brain stem and the area between the brainstem and the cerebellum is called the cerebellopontine angle.

Some of the different structures of the brain seen on scans are the parenchyma consisting of white matter and grey matter, the subarachnoid spaces including the basal cisterns, the ventricular system, the substance of the cerebellum and then the bony vault and skull base surrounding the brain. T1 WI are excellent for demonstrating normal anatomy. In evaluating a patient's radiology, it is important to make sure that you know how many films have been done. A patient may have several sets of films; there may be three CT scan films, one for evaluation of the bone in which only bone windows were done and the brain had been factored out, one where soft tissue had been factored in without contrast and one where soft tissue had been factored in post contrast enhancement. The MRI will usually consist of several types of sequences with T2 WI and pre and post contrast T1 WI being the most common. The MRI will consist of not only axial cuts but also coronal and sagittal cuts. When putting the scans up onto the viewer, look in the right upper corner of each of the small images and identify the name of the patient. Ensure the scan is orientated the correct way around (if the name of the patient is not back to front or upside down, you are correct in your orientation). Ensure that the films you are looking at are for the correct scan date. Then try to find a "c" sign, the word "contrast", "gadolinium" or "gad" on the scan within the small square. This indicates that contrast had been administered.

When reading scans you need to have a system and be methodical. A useful system is to approach the scan from the outside inwards. Therefore, if we look at the large square of film that the scan is printed on, we start at the outside of the film and and look at the survey or scout image. This gives us a general idea of the way that the gantry of the scanner has been angled, by seeing the way that the lines go through the anatomical plane of the head and how many slices have been done. For instance, in the posterior fossa it is usual to do thinner cuts than in the rest of the brain. When presenting a scan you would start by saying "This is a contrasted (or uncontrasted) axial, sagittal or coronal CT/MRI (T1 or T2 weighted) scan of (person's name) done on (date of scan) and the most striking abnormality is ......"
Progressing from the outside of the slice inwards, look firstly at the bone and, if you have a CT scan with bony windows, concentrate on these first. When looking at CT scans, be aware that there are several suture lines in the skull. The most obvious sutures are the lambdoid and the coronal suture. The coronal suture is seen about a third of the way back from the anterior part of the skull and the lambdoid suture is seen in the region of the posterior fossa cuts, see figure 7. MRI sequences are of little or no benefit when evaluating bone.

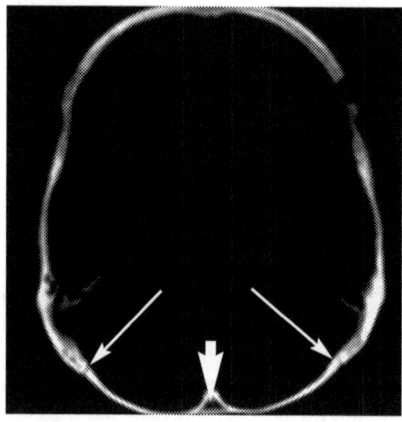

Figure 7. *This is a bone window of an axial CT scan. Both lambdoid sutures are indicated with the thin white arrows and the internal occipital protuberance with the thick white arrow. Note the burrhole in the left frontal region.*

Then, as far as the substance of the cerebrum is concerned, try to look for asymmetry. The sulcal pattern is a useful adjunct in this as a mass lesion in a hemisphere may flatten the sulcal pattern on that side. The sulci can be seen best on the convexity of the brain, at the top half, in the first few cuts from the vertex downwards. When identifying lesions on a scan it is important to be able to describe them. You need to describe whether the lesion is homogenous or not. There might be a central necrotic or cystic component with the lesion having heterogeneous appearance of both solid tumour and cyst or it may be a homogenous (uniform density), solid tumour. Does the lesion have an irregular or regular outline, does it enhance with contrast and is there any associated oedema or mass effect? Having carefully studied the cerebral hemispheres, it is important to then focus on the ventricular system.

Hydrocephalus and ventriculomegaly

Any dilatation of the ventricular system or asymmetry should be noted. When the ventricles are dilated, it may be due to brain atrophy (hydrocephalus ex vacuo) and in this case the sulcal pattern will be enlarged as well as the basal cisterns. Alternatively, it could be due to hydrocephalus, in which case the ventricles become larger but the sulcal pattern and the basal cisterns become smaller due to the compressive effect of the ventricles. It is important to differentiate between communicating and non-communicating hydrocephalus. A basic rule is that if all four the ventricles are large then the ventricles are all communicating with each other and it is therefore communicating hydrocephalus. If there are one or two ventricles that are large and the rest are small then it is non-communicating hydrocephalus. For instance, a colloid cyst of the third ventricle will block off the foramina of Monroe and will cause both lateral ventricles to distend. The fourth ventricle which is not in communication with the lateral ventricles, due to an obstruction at the level of foramen of Monroe, will be normal in size, and this a non-communicating pattern of hydrocephalus. In communicating hydrocephalus, the obstruction is outside of the ventricular system and it can either be because the subarachnoid spaces and cisterns are obliterated, the outlet foramina are obstructed or because there is decreased absorption by the arachnoid villae.

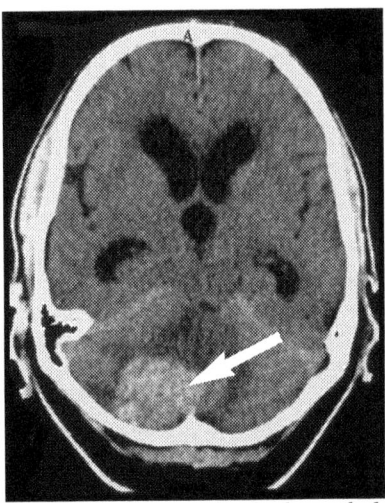

Figure 8. *Obstructive hydrocephalus. This is an uncontrasted axial CT scan. There is a haemorrhage in the posterior fossa (arrow) which is obstructing the fourth ventricle leading to obstructive hydrocephalus with dilatation of both anterior and temporal horns of the lateral ventricles and also dilatation of the third ventricle.*

When evaluating the posterior fossa, it is important to note that the vermis is usually of a different colour than the two cerebellar hemispheres. It can be easy to confuse the normal appearance of the vermis with that of a tumour. In patients presenting after a head injury it is important to evaluate the skull base for fractures. These are seen best on the bony cuts of the CT scan, which should be performed in all traumatic cases.

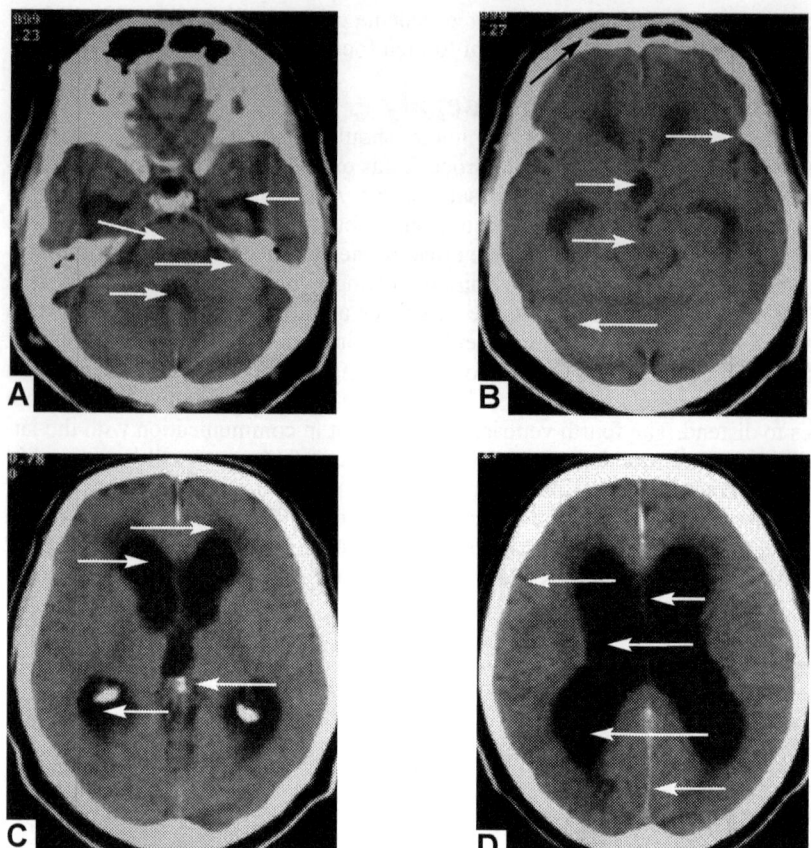

Figure 9. *These are uncontrasted axial CT scans. In these images communicating hydrocephalus is depicted with dilatation of all the ventricles and the arrows are described from top to bottom; A: The top arrow demonstrates the dilated temporal horn of the left lateral ventricle, the next arrow demonstrates the pons, the next arrow demonstrates the left petrous part of the temporal bone and the last arrow shows the dilated fourth ventricle; B: The top arrow demonstrates the frontal air sinus, the next arrow the top part of the sphenoid ridge of the left temporal bone, next arrow demonstrates the dilated third ventricle, the next arrow the midbrain and the last arrow demonstrates the folia of the right cerebellar hemisphere; C: The top arrow demonstrates periventricular lucency due the increased hydrostatic pressure of CSF in the ventricle, the next arrow demonstrates the dilated frontal horn of the right lateral ventricle, the next arrow demonstrates the pineal gland and the next arrow the trigone of the right lateral ventricle containing choroid plexus; D: The top arrow depicts a cerebral sulcus, the next the septum pellucidum, the next demonstrates the body of the right lateral ventricle, the next the occipital horn of the right lateral ventricle and the last arrow demonstrates the falx cerebri.*

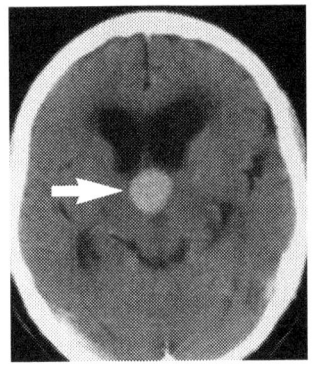

Figure 10. *Obstructive hydrocephalus. A colloid cyst of the third ventricle blocks both the foramina of Monroe bilaterally leading to obstructive hydrocephalus of the lateral ventricles.*

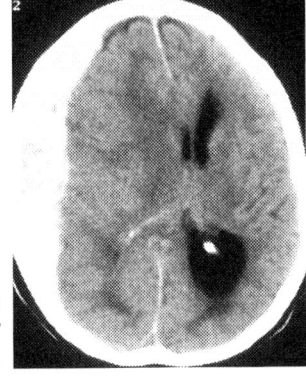

Figure 11. *Obstructive hydrocephalus. This is an uncontrasted axial CT scan. The acute subdural haemorrhage on the right has caused midline shift and trapped the frontal and occipital horns of the left lateral ventricle leading to dilatation and hydrocephalus.*

Trauma

A CT scan is the preferred investigation for cranial trauma. It does not require MR compatible ventilators or instruments, is simple, fast and widely available. The images are very sensitive for acute haemorrhage as well as cerebral oedema. CT scans are also the preferred imaging modality for evaluating bone and is an excellent tool for diagnosing fractures of the skull base, skull vault and facial bones. In trauma, the main categories of pathology are skull fractures, diffuse brain injury, intracerebral haemorrhages and extra-axial haemorrhages.

Skull fractures

The telltale sign of a skull fracture on a CT scan is usually overlying soft tissue swelling or disruption of the soft tissue with gas in the tissue. Fractures may be linear or depressed, comminuted or simple. Depressed fractures are frequently associated with dural tears and underlying intracerebral haemorrhages. Base of skull fractures may be difficult to identify, as they can often be hairline cracks. Fluid in the mastoid air cells or in the frontal sinus (opacification of the sinus) is frequently an indication of a skull base fracture with an associated dural tear and CSF leak. Intracranial air is another indication of a dural tear.

Diffuse brain injury

Diffuse brain injury (DBI) is part of a wide spectrum ranging from concussion to severe diffuse axonal injury. The hallmark of diffuse brain injury is pinpoint haemorrhage. These occur due to acceleration -deceleration and rotational forces imparted to the brain with subsequent tears in the white matter tracts, leading to pin point haemorrhages. They are usually found at the grey – white matter interface.

There are three grades of DBI:

Grade 1 – diffuse point bleeds throughout the brain.
Grade 2 – as above with point bleeds in the corpus callosum and
Grade 3 – as grade 2 with point bleeds in the dorsal mid-brain.

These 3 grades correlate well with prognosis and mid-brain haemorrhages are usually associated with a poor prognosis. Acute subdural haematomas are frequently associated with DBI as the rotational forces and acceleration - deceleration forces can lead to the draining veins suspended between the dura and the cortical surface being torn with subsequent haemorrhage into the subdural space.

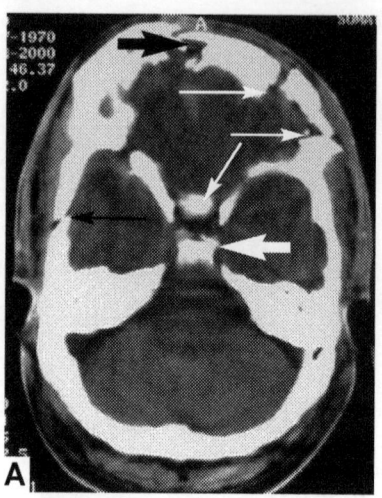 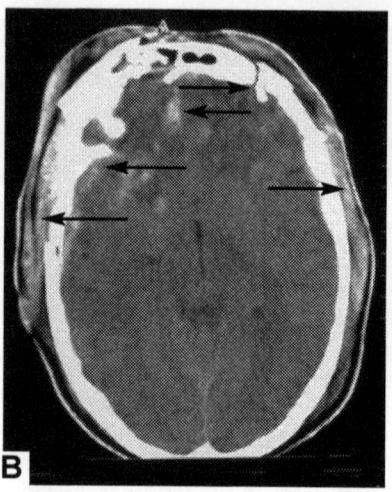

Figure 12. *These are uncontrasted axial CT scans. These images depict severe cranial trauma. A: The top 3 arrows depict a comminuted fracture of the frontal bone involving the frontal air sinus, the lower black arrow depicts a fracture of the right temporal bone, the angled arrow shows the tuberculum sellae and the thick white arrow the dorsum sellae B: The top arrow demonstrates a linear fracture of the frontal bone, the next demonstrates frontal lobe haemorrhagic contusions, the next a thin acute subdural haematoma and the last two arrows demonstrate extracranial soft tissue swelling secondary to traumatic impacts.*

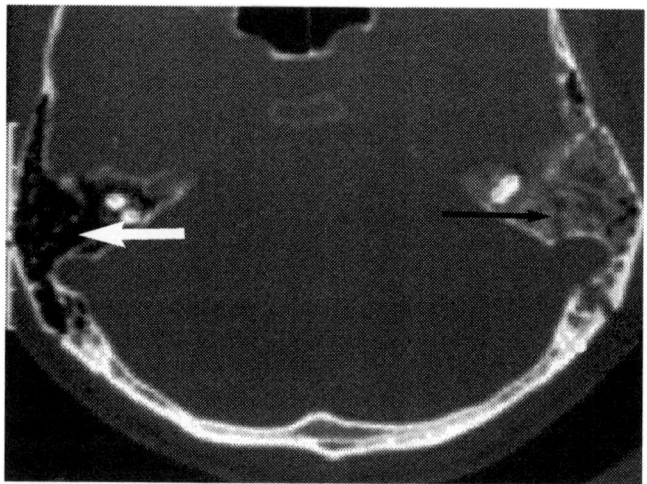

Figure 13. *This is the bone window of an axial CT scan. The black arrow depicts a transverse fracture of the petrous part of the temporal bone. This base of skull fracture has opacified the mastoid air cells on the left. The normal black appearance of the right sided mastoid air cells (thick arrow) is because they are filled with air whereas the white opacified air cells on the right are filled with fluid secondary to the fracture.*

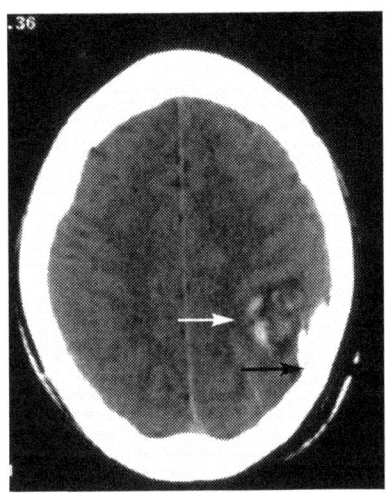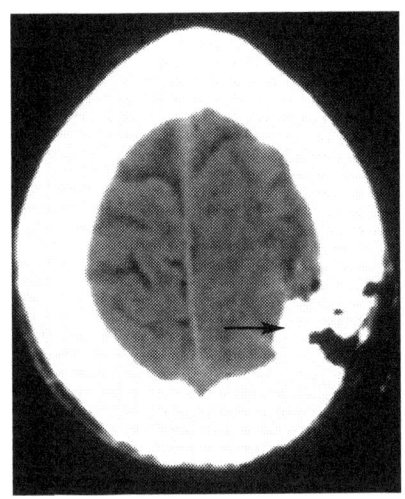

Figure 14. *These are uncontrasted axial CT scans. A comminuted, depressed fracture is depicted on these two axial slices (black arrows) with an underlying haemorrhagic contusion (white arrow). This is a typical example of focal brain trauma.*

Diffuse Injury Grade	CT appearance	Mortality
I	Normal CT scan	9.6%
II	Basal cisterns not effaced and midline shift < 5mm	13.5%
III	Cisterns compressed or absent and midline shift < 5mm	34%
IV	Shift > 5mm but no mass lesion of >25 cm^3 present	56.2%

Table 1. *The Marshall classification.*
(Marshall LF, Bowers-Marshall S, Klauber MR et al. A new classification of head injury based on computerised tomography. J Neurosurg 75 (Suppl):S14-20, 1991)

Intracerebral haemorrhage
We frequently see coup and contrecoup injuries where the impact side (coup side) as well as the opposite side (contrecoup side) demonstrates traumatic brain damage. This may for instance happen when a person falls onto the back of their head. The patient will have focal soft tissue swelling over the occiput with some focus of pathology there, frequently an intracerebral haemorrhage with some associated subarachnoid haemorrhage. Also the brain then moves forward and rubs over the rough surface of the orbital roof in the anterior cranial fossa and the frontal lobe poles impact against the inner skull leading to bifrontal contusions. There are frequently associated bitemporal contusions as the anterior poles of the temporal lobes collide with the sphenoid ridge, which forms the anterior border of the middle cranial fossa. These are devastating injuries and with longterm sequelae. These contusions quite often "blossom" as they enlarge and have associated oedema, usually about a week after the injury. Other intracerebral haemorrhages, called haemorrhagic contusions, can be larger versions of the pinpoint bleeds in diffuse brain injury and are caused by the same mechanism.

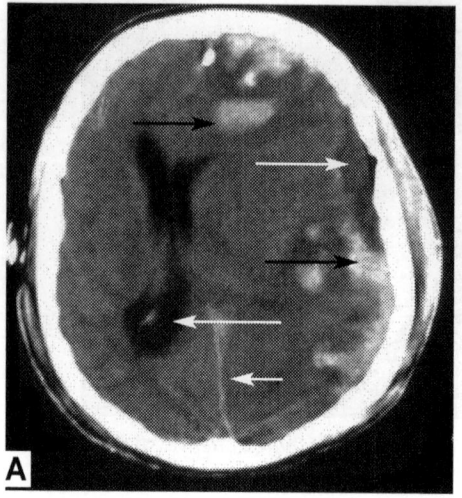 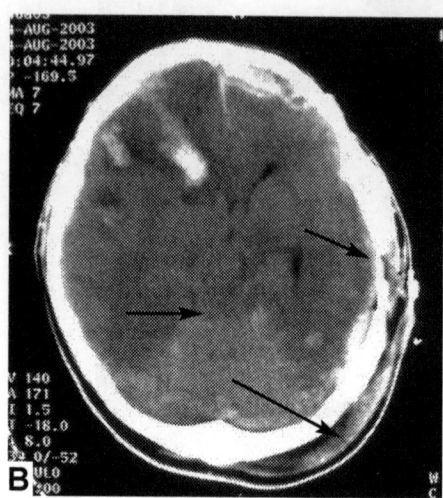

Figure 15. *These are uncontrasted axial CT scans. Both images depict severe diffuse brain injury. Note how on the left the hemisphere has swollen up and is herniating across the midline. A: The top arrow depicts a haemorrhagic contusion and several of these can be seen throughout both hemispheres, the next arrow demonstrates a hyperacute component of an acute subdural haematoma where the blood is so fresh that it has not yet had the time to clot and become hyperdense. It is important not to confuse this with a chronic subdural haematoma which has the same density. The next arrow demonstrates the clotted component of the acute subdural haematoma, the next arrow demonstrates the trapped ventricles due to midline shift and the last arrows demonstrates a parafalcine acute subdural haematoma. B: The top arrow shows a skull fracture. The next arrow demonstrates obliteration of the basal cisterns due to brain swelling. The last arrow demonstrates the widespread soft tissue swelling secondary to focal impacts. In this case the haemorrhagic contusions, acute subdural haematoma and parafalcine subdural haematoma point towards a diffuse brain injury with acceleration-deceleration and rotational forces and the skull fracture to a focal, impact type injury. This is typical for motor vehicle accidents where there is a combination of these mechanisms of injury.*

Extra-axial collections

Subdural and extradural collections may be difficult to tell apart. Subdural collections are usually craggy, irregularly shaped and depress the underlying brain. Epidural (extradural) haemorrhages are bicrescentic or biconvex lesions that strip the dura away from the bone. On CT scans both are white in the acute phase. In the hyperacute phase, before the blood has had a chance to clot, these lesions are darker than the brain and hypodense. Following the acute phase, the blood lyses and turns into deoxyhaemoglobin and bilirubin and it becomes more serous. The colour on CT scans changes to become more grey and eventually it becomes dark, very much the same density as the CSF. This happens over a couple of weeks. There is definite clinical significance in differentiating between a subdural and extradural haemorrhage. A subdural haemorrhage may sometimes continue to bleed but far more so, extradural haematomas have the propensity to do this. This gives rise to 'the talk and die' phenomenon where patients arrive in the hospital awake (the lucid interval) but then subsequently deteriorate due to ongoing haemorrhage from the ruptured vessel on the dural surface leading to increased haematoma formation and brain compression.

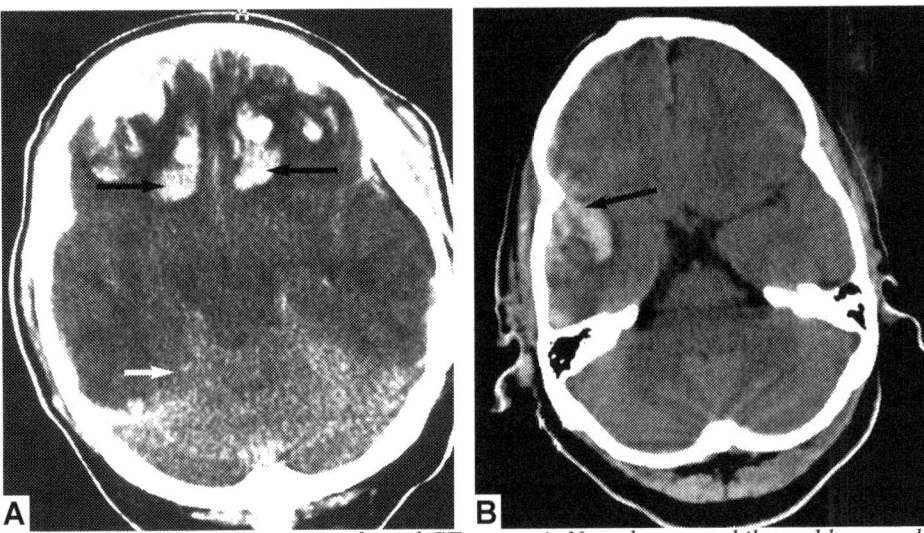

Figure 16. *These are uncontrasted axial CT scans. A: Note the severe bilateral haemorrhagic contusions (black arrows) and note the difference in density between the area of the tentorium cerebelli and the rest of the brain (white arrow). It can be difficult to tell whether this is due to ischaemia in the frontal and temporal lobes or is just the different imaging characteristics of the dura (tentorium cerebelli) and the brain parenchyma. These contusions are usually caused when the brain moves forward over the rough surface of the anterior cranial fossa; B: The movement of the brain cause the parenchyma of the frontal and temporal lobes adjacent to the Sylvian fissure to collide with the sphenoid ridge of the temporal bone, causing haemorrhagic contusions and in this case a small acute subdural haematoma (black arrow).*

When evaluating these lesions it is important to note their location, how big they are and what their effects are on the brain. When reporting these lesions, especially to a senior colleague, state the location of the haemorrhage and on how many cuts it can be seen on the CT scan as this indicates the total volume of the clot. CT scans are usually performed in 7 or 8mm cuts (the vertical distance between the slices) in the supratentorial area and therefore a haemorrhage that can be seen on 7 cuts is between 5-6cms high. When this is combined with the thickness of the clot you can get an estimate of how large it is. A haematoma 1 or 2 cm wide that can be seen on 4 or 5 cuts would be judged to be a large haematoma. It is sometimes difficult to visually separate the haematoma from the bone (since both are white) and if looking at the scans on the CT workstation it can be useful to change the settings of the scan (ask the radiographer to help you) and this frequently demonstrates the interface between the bone and the blood. Using Hounsfield units are also useful. It is important to look at the effect on the underlying brain and a midline shift of 5mm or more is significant. An extra-axial collection in the temporal lobe has much more clinical effect than a collection on the convexity as the temporal lobe is situated adjacent to the midbrain and even small haematomas can cause compression of the midbrain. It is easy to see the edge of the tentorium cerebelli at the medial border of the temporal lobe and it is possible to see herniation of the brain tissue (uncus) through this hiatus with subsequent compression of the brainstem. Acute extradural haematomas usually result from injury to the anterior or posterior branches of the middle meningeal artery. However, fractures associated with venous sinuses can also lead to extradural haematomas caused by a venous bleed rather than an arterial source. Venous extradural haematomas are more common in children. Subdural haematomas can also be interhemispheric or be found on the surface of the tentorium cerebelli.

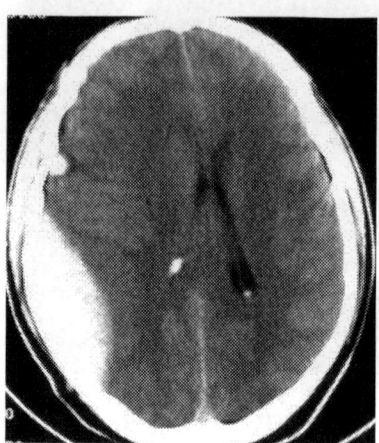

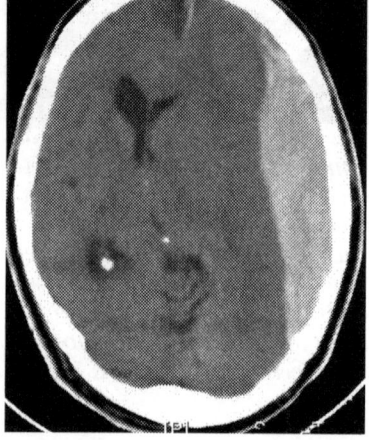

Figure 17. *This is an uncontrasted axial CT scan and it demonstrates an acute extradural haematoma with typical biconvex shape. This is because the dura is stripped away from the brain by the haematoma. These haematomas usually do not cross the suture lines.*

Figure 18. *This is an uncontrasted axial CT scan and it demonstrates an acute subdural collection with typical crescenteric shape. Note the marked midline shift as in figure 17 above.*

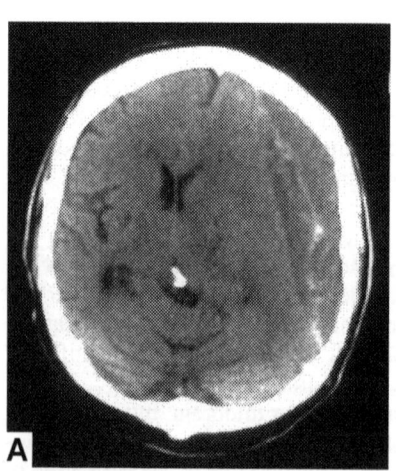

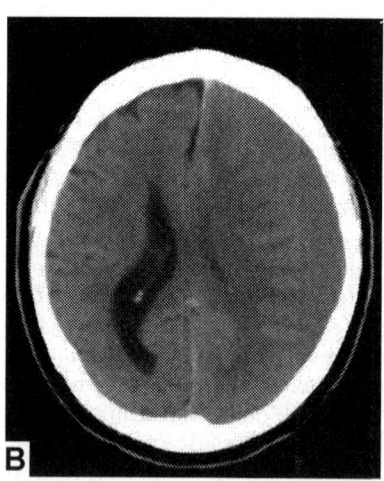

Figure 19. *These are uncontrasted axial CT scans. A: This chronic subdural haematoma is hypodense to brain. B: In this scan the subdural haematoma is isodense to brain making it very difficult to diagnose. It is the midline shift in these cases that make the diagnosis. The most difficult scenario is that of bilateral isodense subdural haematomas where there is no midline shift. In these cases, the ventricles will usually appear compressed and the basal cisterns and the sulci are also compressed.*

Brain tumours

Brain tumours can be either primary or secondary (metastasis). The administration of contrast medium greatly improves the CT sensitivity and specificity for tumour diagnosis. Enhancement with contrast may either represent blood-brain barrier breakdown or tumour neo-vascularity. Because of disruption of the normal cyto architecture in brain tumours, the blood-brain barrier does not remain intact and this allows seepage of contrast out of the vascular system. Similarly, the fast growing tissue of malignant tumours requires new blood vessels to feed the rapidly growing cells and this will lead to contrast enhancement at the area of the tumour. This is because tumours have more blood vessels and therefore more contrast density/intensity than the surrounding normal brain. Tumours are divided into intra-axial (within the neural axis that is the parenchyma of the brain or the spinal cord limited by the pia mater) and extra-axial tumours (outside of the neural axis and therefore outside the brain parenchyma and pia mater).

There are glial and non glial brain tumours. High grade lesions generally tend to enhance with contrast and have a poor prognosis where low grade lesionms tend not to enhance and have a better prognosis. Glial tumours include tumours from astrocytes, oligodendrocytes and ependymal cells. There are also tumnours that arise from the meninges and these tend to enhance strongly. Lymphomas, tumours arising from pluripotent stem cells and tumours arising from blood vessels are part of the spectrum. Tumours are described based on their consistency, shape, enhancement and position. Metastatic tumours are frequently multiple. Cysts are homogenous, dark areas on CT scans and are white on T2 WI and dark on T1 WI. They may have associated nodules if they are tumour cysts. Abscesses are circular cystic areas with strong enhancement. They are frequently in a paraventricular location or in association with cranial air sinuses.

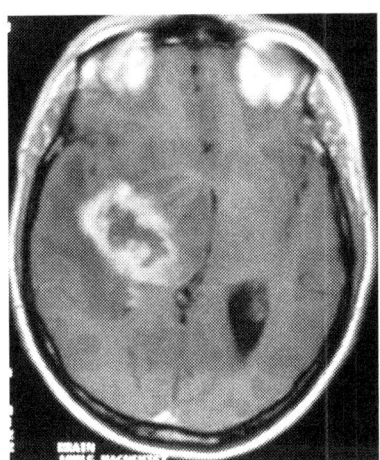
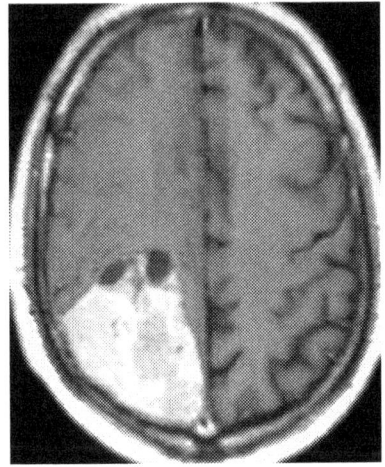

Figure 20. *These are contrast enhanced axial T1 weighted MR scans. A: This is atypical picture of a glioblastoma multiforma which is the highest grade of glial tumour. B: This is a typical picture of a meningioma, which arises from the meninges and therefore outside of the substance of the brain.*

Figure 21. *This is a contrast enhanced axial T1 weighted MR scan and it demonstrates a cyst in the posterior fossa with an associated enhancing mural nodule. This is a hemangioblastoma which is a benign condition.*

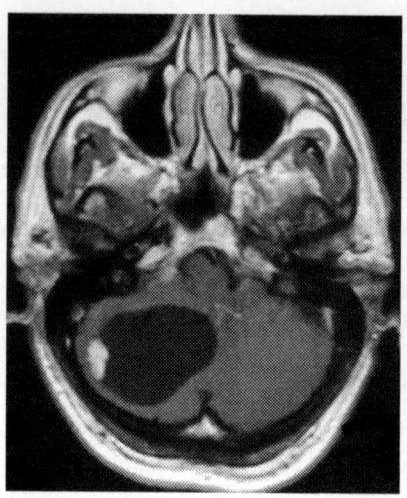

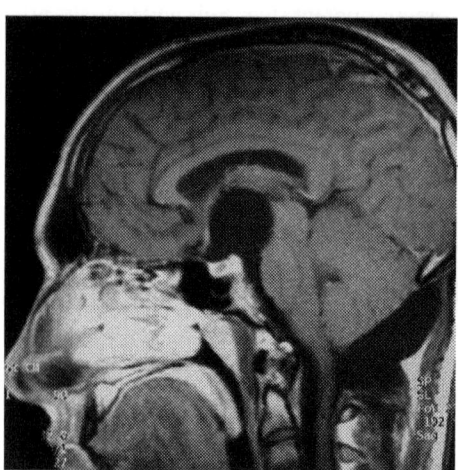

Figure 22. *This is an unenhanced sagittal T1 wieghted MR scan and it demonstrates this prepontine arachnoid cyst which is an incidental developmental abnormality of the leptomeninges causing a local obstruction of, and collection of CSF in a cyst.*

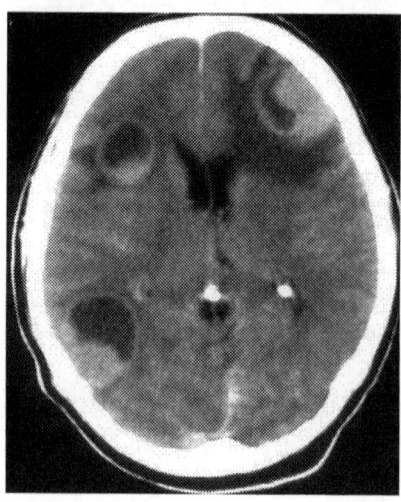

Figure 23. *These multiple enhancing lesions are typical of metastatic lesions. The prognosis for these lesions are poor. That is because there are usually several lesions that are smaller and not visible on imaging. Treatment would consist primarily of radiotherapy with surgical excision of superficial lesion. This is a axial, contrast enhanced CT scan.*

Figure 24. *These images (unenhanced axila CT scans) all demonstrate subarachnoid haemorrhage. The top scan demonstrates the following: The two black arrows demonstrate blood in the Sylvian fissures, the top white arrow demonstrates blood in the basal cisterns and the next white arrow demonstrates dilated temporal horns which is an early sign of hydrocephalus. The bottom scan demonstrates the following: The top arrow demonstrates blood in the occipital horns of the lateral ventricle, the next arrow demonstrates blood in the left Sylvian fissure and the next two demonstrate dilated temporal horns of the lateral ventricles.*

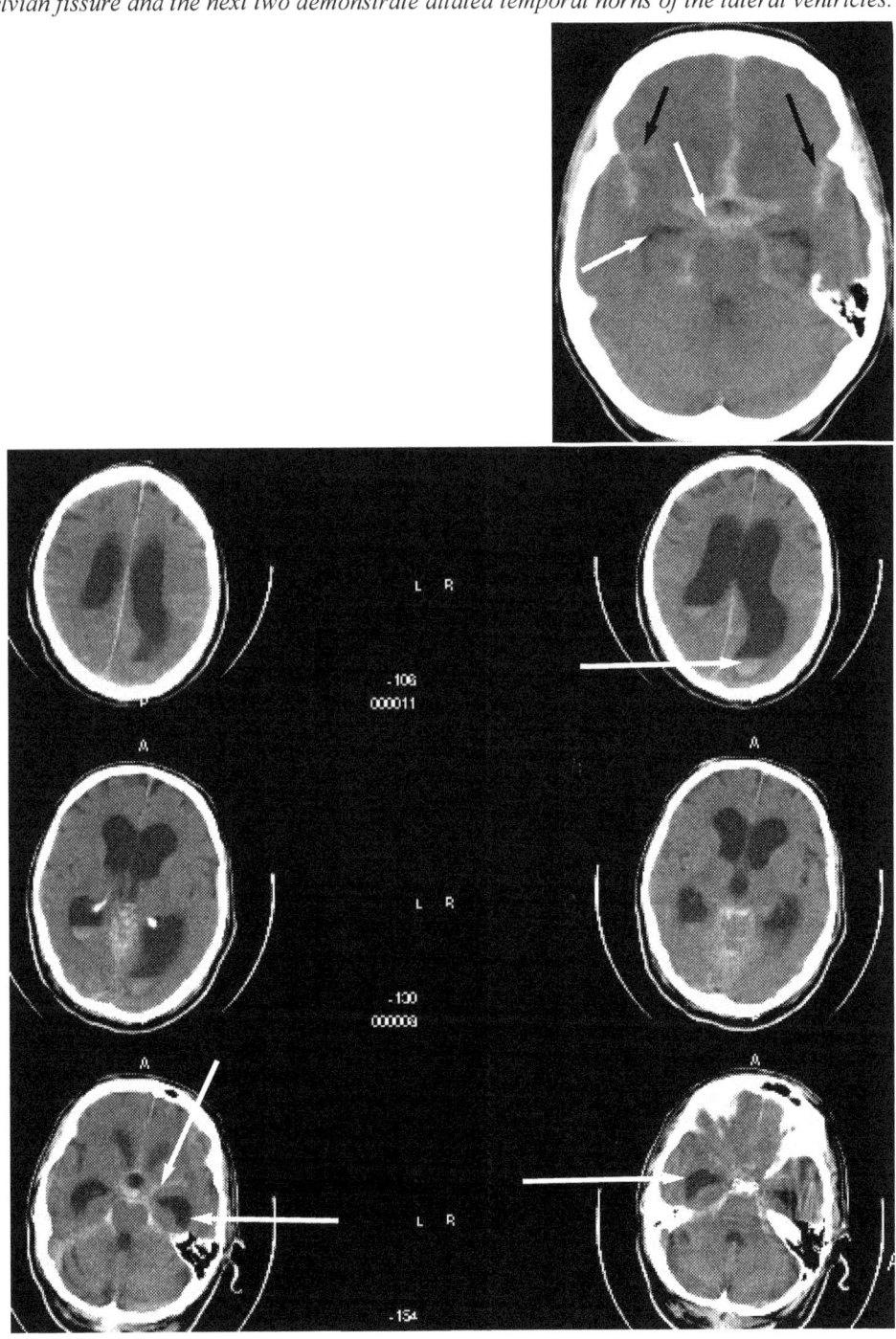

Figure 25. These are unenhanced axial CT scans. The top image demonstrates a left middle cerebral artery infarction. The bottom scan demonstrates a huge intraparenchymal haemorrhage that has broken through into the ventricular system.

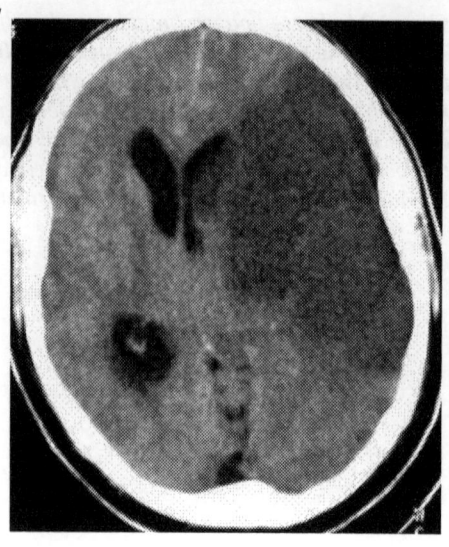

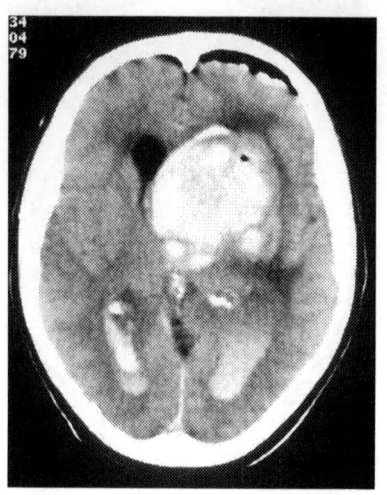

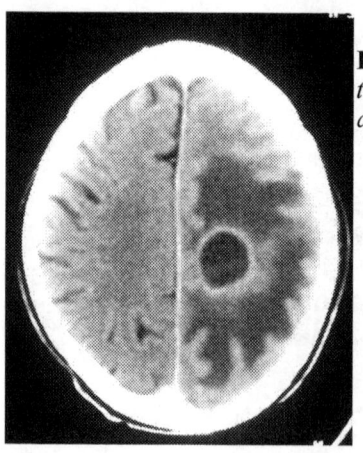

Figure 26. This contrast enhanced axial CT scan shows the typical ring enhancing appearance of an intracerebral abscess.

4

SPINAL IMAGING

Contents

Normal appearances of spinal MR imaging
Clearing C-spine X-rays following trauma
Degenerative conditions
Spinal tumours
Cysts
Infection

Normal appearances of the spine on MR imaging

Vertebrae

Vertebral bodies are hyperintense compared to spinal cord on T1 WI with the marrow (containing fat) being more intense than the rest of the vertebra. The vertebrae are of a slightly higher intensity that the intervertebral discs on T1 WI. The hallmark of pathology in vertebrae is a decrease on T1 WI and an increase of intensity on T2 WI due to the increased water content associated with most pathology and the displacement of the normal marrow.

Neural foramina

When evaluating sagittal MR scans as in figure 1, the scout view will orientate you as to whether the image is to the right or the left of the midline. The upper portion of the neural foramen contains fatty connective tissue with the nerve root located in the inferior portion of the foramen. The nerve root will be displaced in lateral disc protrusions and may be displaced upwards, displacing the fatty tissue.

Intervertebral disc

Healthy discs in young patients have a high water content and therefore are hypointense on T1 WI and relatively hyperintense on T2 WI. As patients get older, the discs dehydrate or they may dehydrate secondary to pathological processes, becoming relatively hypointense on T2 WI compared to normal discs. The annulus fibrous appears as a hypointense signal on T1WI and T2 WI.

Spinal cord

All neural tissues demonstrate intermediate signal intensity (gray) on both T1 and T2 WI. CSF demonstrates hypointensity on T1 WI and is hyperintense on T2 WI.

Clearing C-spine X-rays following trauma

The following three views are essential and mandatory:
Lateral c-spine film demonstrating the C7-T1 junction clearly and demonstrating the upper border of T1. If this is not possible with a normal lateral film, then a swimmers view should be performed (one arm above the head).
A-P view
Open mouth view demonstrating the odontoid process.

The following sequence is useful in clearing the cervical spine:
Alignment – Assess the alignment of the anterior vertebral line, the posterior vertebral line and the spinolaminar line. More than 3.5 mm subluxation is abnormal. At C2/C3 there may be a normal physiological subluxation of up to 3mm, especially in children. Subluxation of up to 50% of the width of the vertebral body signifies unifacet dislocation and a subluxation of more than this signifies a bifacet dislocation, which is usually accompanied by widening of the interspinous spaces.
Angulation – angulation of more than 11 degrees between two adjacent vertebrae is indicative of a fracture or ligamentous injury and potential instability.
The diameter of the spinal canal – anything less than 14 mm is indicative of impending spinal cord compression.
Examination of the pre vertebral soft tissue shadow - from C1 to C4 the soft tissue should be maximally half the width of a vertebral body and below C4 it should be maximally equal to the width of a vertebral body (5mm at C2 and 17 - 22 mm at C6).
The distance between the skull base and the atlas should not exceed 5mm as this can be indicative of atlanto – occipital dissociation.
The vertebral bodies should be examined to ascertain that there are no compression fractures or burst fractures.
The intervertebral discs are not visible on plain x-rays or CT scans but they can be examined by looking at the disc spaces between the vertebrae which demonstrate the anatomy of the (invisible) discs. Therefore a narrowing of one disc space will imply that there has been compression, and possibly herniation, of an intervertebral disc. If there is an associated neurological deficit without a fracture or dislocation, an MR scan will demonstrate the anatomy of the disc and any related prolapse.
The odontoid peg should be examined on the open mouth view for fractures. The vertical line that separates the front teeth must not be confused with a fracture. On the lateral c-spine view there should not be more than 3mm between the dens and the atlas (atlanto-dens interval). More than this implies injury to the transverse ligament and more than 5mm implies disruption of this ligament.

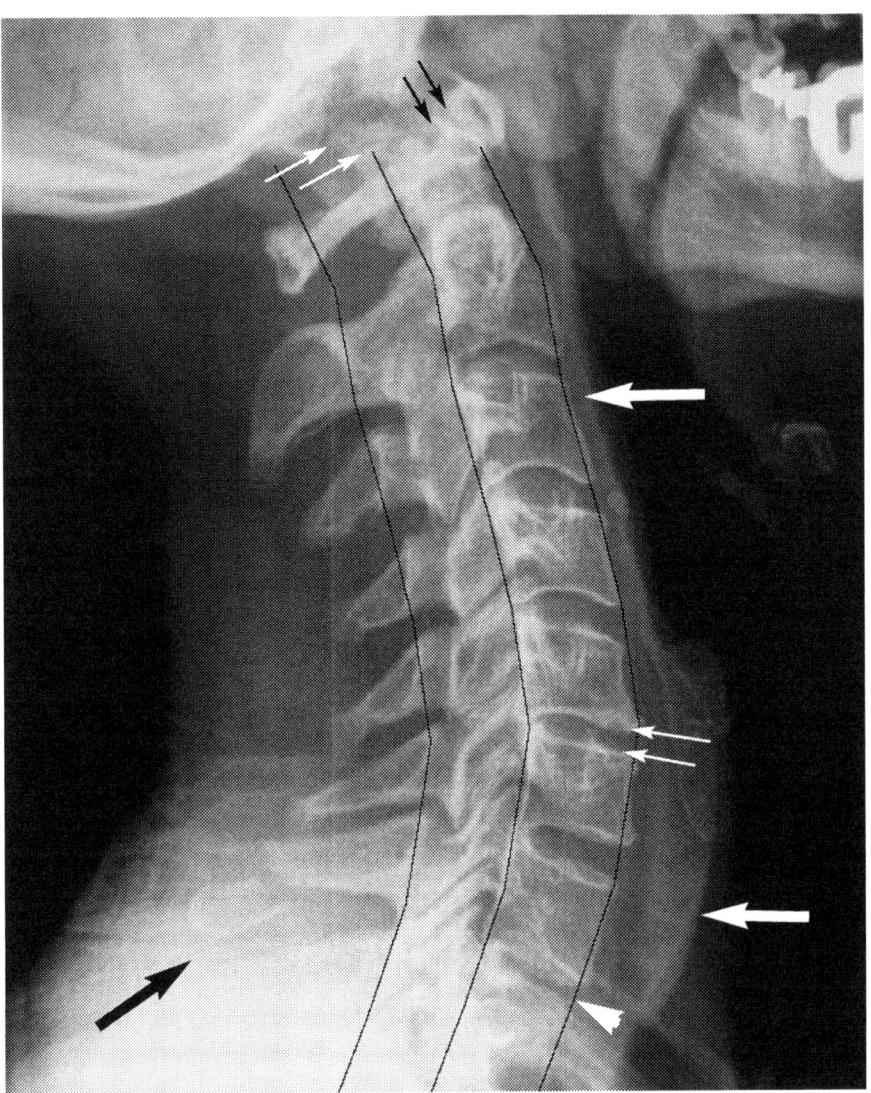

Figure 1. *This image depicts a lateral cervical spine x-ray. The two thin black arrows at the skull base demonstrates the atlanto-dens interval which should not exceed 3mm. The two thin white arrows demonstrate the space between the top of the atlas and the base of the skull which should not exceed 5mm. The top thick white arrow demonstrates the pre vertebral soft tissue shadow from C1 to C4 and the bottom thick white arrow the soft tissue below C4. The soft tissue from C1 to C4 should be maximally half the width of a vertebral body and below C4 it should be maximally equal to the width of a vertebral body (5mm at C2 and 17 - 22 mm at C6). The bottom two thin white arrows point toward a narrowed C5/6 disc space. MRI confirmed a C5/6 disc prolapse. The thick white arrow head points at the top edge of T1 which must always be seen. The thick black arrow points toward a clay shoveler's fracture (avulsion fracture of the tip of the spinous process). Note the three lines (anterior vertebral line, the posterior vertebral line and the spinolaminar line) demonstrating the alignment of the cervical spine.*

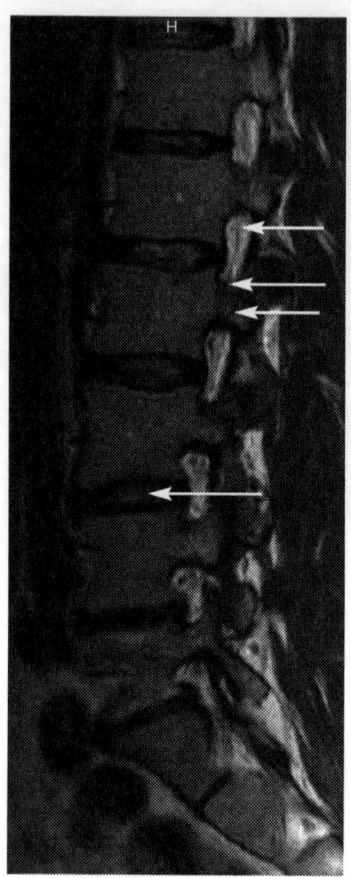

Figure 2. *This is a sagittal T2 WI of the lumbosacral spine. This image is taken off the midline, and in this case to the right of the spinal canal, and demonstrates the neural foramina, which are white due to the fatty tissue contained within them. The top arrow points toward the top of a neural foramen and the next arrow to the bottom. Note that this arrow points directly at the nerve as it lies in the inferior part of the foramen. The third arrow points directly at a pedicle. The last arrow points at an intervertebral disc.*

Degenerative conditions
Rheumatoid arthritis
CT scanning may demonstrate C1/2 subluxation, cranial settling and dens erosions. MRI may demonstrate pannus formation and acquired spinal stenosis. Plain flexion and extension images as well as MR in flexion and extension are invaluable to demonstrate dynamic subluxations.

Spinal stenosis
Spinal stenosis is either congenital or acquired. Sagittal T2 WI demonstrates spinal stenosis well but the most useful image is the axial T2 WI. In the cervical spine, anterior compression of the spinal cord can be caused by prolapsed discs, osteophytic bars, ossification of the posterior longitudinal ligament, subluxation of the vertebrae and vertebral compression fractures. Posterior and lateral compression can be caused by hypertrophy of the ligamentum flavum and the facet joints. Damage to the cord is shown as hyperintensity on the T2 WI. In the lumbar spine the classic trefoil shape can be seen with the round canal taking on a triangular shape. There is usually encroachment due to facet joint hypertrophy as well as thickened ligamentum flavum. Added stenosis is caused by degrees of vertebral body subluxation and plain film extension and flexion views are important in identifying whether this is stable or not.

Disc herniation (prolapse)
The best images to evaluate the presence of disc herniation are the T2 WI as the CSF, being brilliantly white, contrasts well with the rest of the tissue and demonstrating a disc protrusion is easier than on T1WI where the intensity of the tissues are frequently quite similar. The best approach is to look at the sagittal T2 WI and pinpoint the pathology. Then use the axial T2 WI to evaluate the extent of the neural compromise. The T1 WI are good for evaluating the intervertebral foramina and looking at fine detail of the nervous structures. The sagittal and coronal images are useful for evaluating the lateral elements.

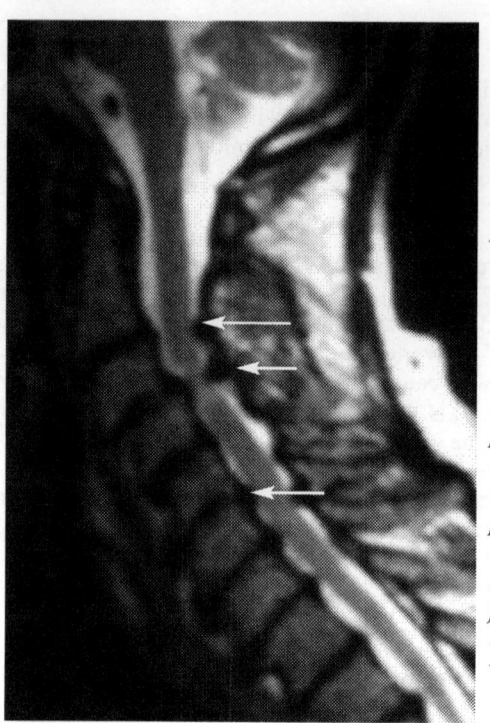

Figure 3. *This is a sagittal T2 WI of the cervical spine in a patient with severe cervical spondylosis and clinical quadri spasticity. The top arrow is pointing at a thickened area of ligamentum flavum, as is the next arrow down. The third arrow points toward anterior compression from a disc-osteophyte complex. Note how this patient has both severe anterior and posterior compression of the spinal cord. The intervertebral discs have associated bony osteophytes which are hard and require extensive drilling at the time of surgery. The decision as to whether a decompression is done from an anterior or posterior approach is based on where the compression is and how many levels are affected. Up to three levels may be decompressed from anterior with anterior cervical discectomies or corpectomies. A posterior approach via laminectomy is usually performed for extensive disease. Flexion and extension X-rays are useful to decide whether fusion is required at the same time.*

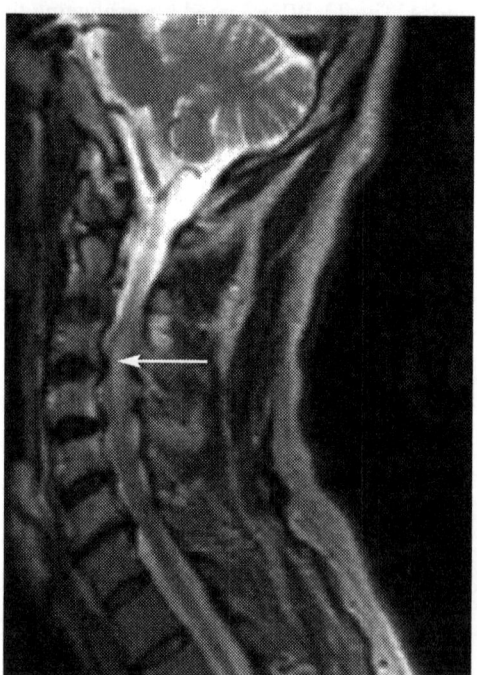

Figure 4. *This sagittal T2 WI of the cervical spine in a different patient from above, also demonstrates severe cervical spondylosis. The arrow is pointing towards associated signal change in the cord, which is a poor prognostic sign.*

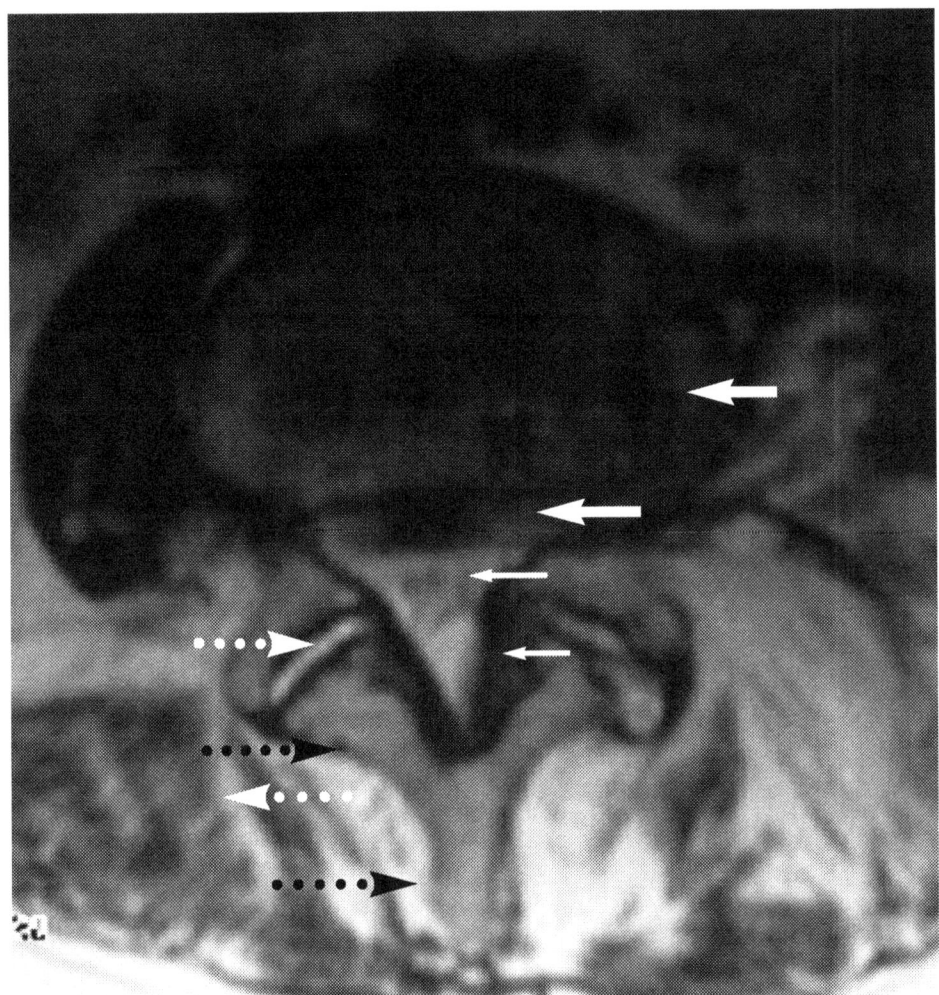

Figure 5. *This is an axial T2 WI of the lumbar spine demonstrating spinal stenosis. The top thick white arrow demonstrates the intervertebral disc. The next thick white arrow demonstrates a broad, flat central disc prolapse. The top thin white arrow demonstrates the compressed cauda equina, which takes on a trefoil shape. The bottom thin white arrow demonstrates the thickened and hypertrophied ligamentum flavum that is a main contributing factor in spinal stenosis. The top dashed white arrow demonstrates the facet joint, the bottom dashed white arrow demonstrates the paraspinal muscles, the top dashed black arrow demonstrates the lamina on the right-hand side and bottom dashed black arrow demonstrates the spinous process.*

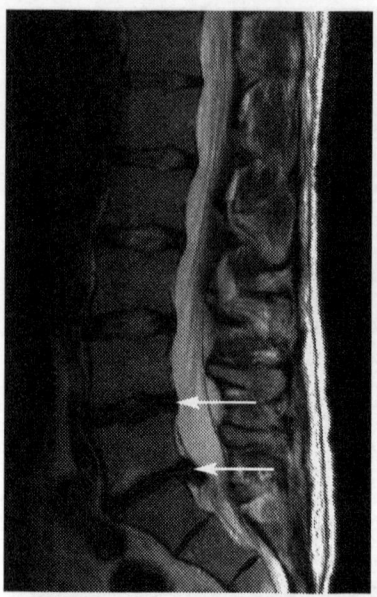
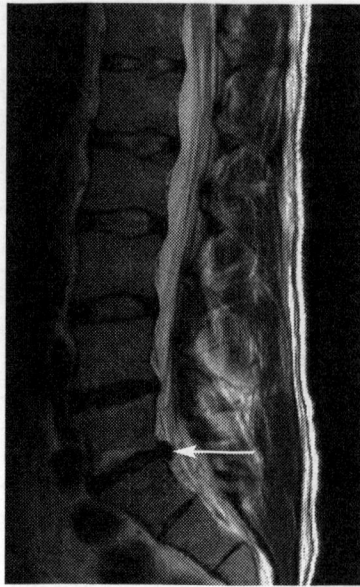
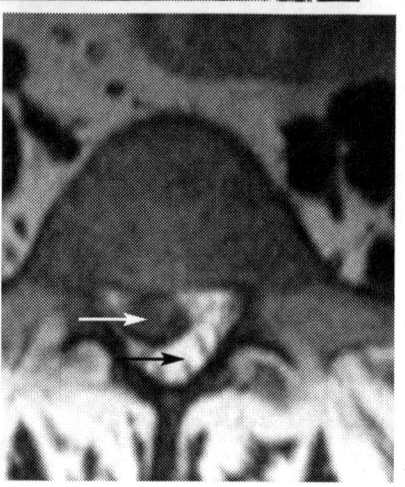

Figure 6. *The top images are sagittal T2 WI and the image on the left is an axial T2 WI of the same patient. The top arrow on the top left image demonstrates a degenerative intervertebral disc. Note how the intensity has changed from the normal intervertebral discs above it. This lower intensity is due to a lower water content of this damaged disc. The next arrow down shows a large downward extrusion of an intervertebral disc. The image top right is an image slightly towards the right of the midline compared to the image on the left. Note how the herniated segment appears smaller. This is because this is a mostly central disc prolapse as is demonstrated in the image on the left by the white arrow. The black arrow demonstrates the cauda equina which is compressed by the disc fragment.*

Spinal tumours

Extradural compartment

Primary tumours
  Bony tumours and cartilage producing tumours of the spine
  Lymphoproliferative tumours
        Solitary plasmacytoma
        Multiple myeloma
Metastatic tumours (prostate, breast adenocarcinoma, lung adenocarcinoma, renal cell carcinoma and gastric carcinoma)

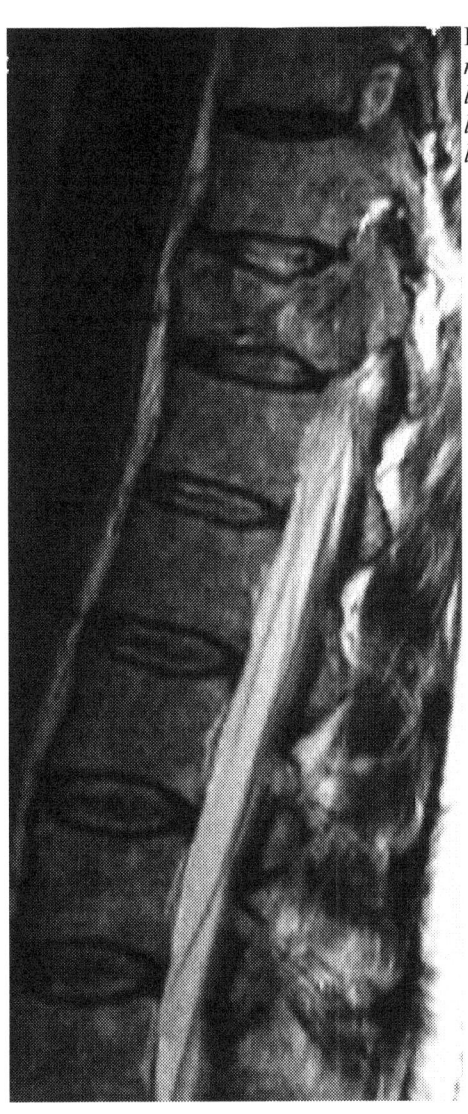

Figure 7. *This is a sagittal T12WI of the thoracic spine which demonstrates a metastatic lesion. It is common for the vertebrae to collapse. Note the sparing of the relatively avascular intervertebral discs.*

Intradural, extramedullary compartment

Meningioma
Schwannoma
Myxopapillary ependymoma (arises in the conus medullaris or filum terminale)

Intramedullary compartment

Ependymoma (55% of intramedullary tumours)
Astrocytoma (30% of intramedullary tumours)
Paraganglioma
Haemangioblastoma

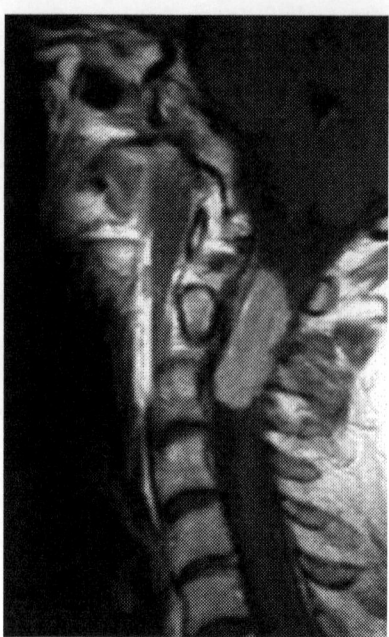 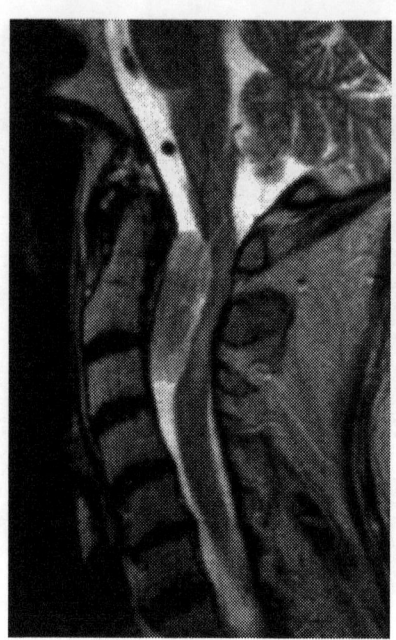

Figure 8. *The image on the top left is a sagittal contrast enhanced T1 WI of the cervical spine and the image top right is a sagittal T2 WI of the cervical spine. Both demonstrate a meningioma. Note how the meningioma is hyperintense to spinal cord following contrast enhancement and hyperintense to cord on the T2 WI. On T1 WI pre contrast these lesions are usually iso/hypointense to the tissue of the spinal cord. The image on the left is a sagittal T1 WI with contrast enhancement demonstrating a meningioma in the thoracic spinal canal.*

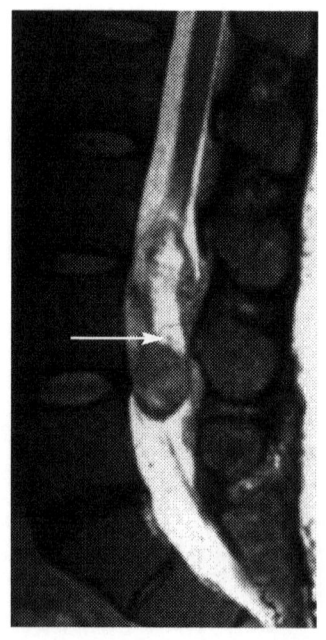

Figure 9. *This sagittal T2 WI of the lumbosacral spine demonstrates a myxopapillary ependymoma of the conus medullaris. Note the heterogeneous appearance and the hyperintense cyst fluid (arrow). This lesion expands the cord circumferentialy outwards.*

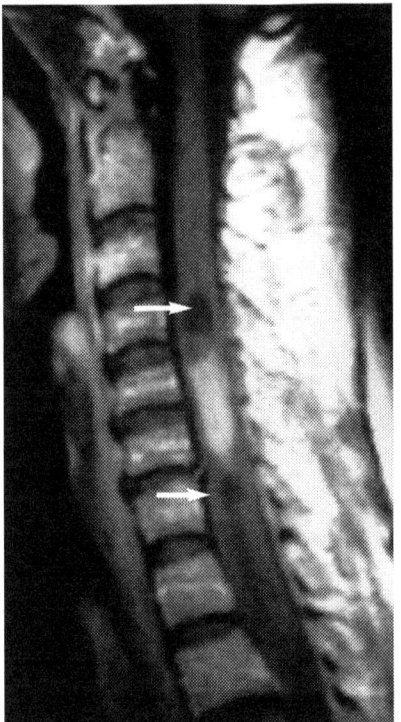 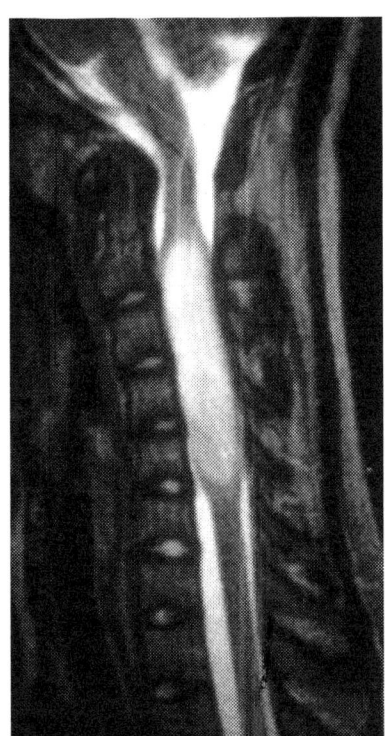

Figure 10. *The image on the left is a sagittal contrast enhanced T1 WI of the cervical spine that demonstrates an ependymoma. Note the two polar cysts as demonstrated by the two arrows. The lesion enhances homogeneously and intensely with contrast. The image on the right is a sagittal T2 WI of the cervical spine and demonstrates an ependymoma. It is homogeneous and hyperintense with good demarcation and is seen to expand the cord.*

Cysts
Arachnoid cyst
Dermoid cyst (located in midline)
Epidermoid cyst (located in midline)
Perineural cyst (Tarlov cyst)
Synovial cyst
Neurenteric cyst

Infection
Osteomyelitis
Discitis
Epidural empyema (abscess)
Tuberculosis of the spine
Infection with *mycobacterium tuberculosis* starts in the vertebra or adjacent endplate and its hallmark is destruction of the vertebra and gibbus formation with collapse of the vertebra, whilst the integrity of the disc is maintained until quite late in the disease. On x-ray vertebral involvement with erosion kyphosis, with mostly involvement of the vertebrae and sparing the posterior elements is seen. There is frequently some soft tissue involvement with calcification. CT scans are quite useful in delineating the extent of the disease and demonstrating bony involvement and bony sequestra. MR may demonstrate as associated cold psoas abscess. Typically, the intervertebral disc is spared with the gibbus hypointense on T1 WI and hyperintense on T2 WI.

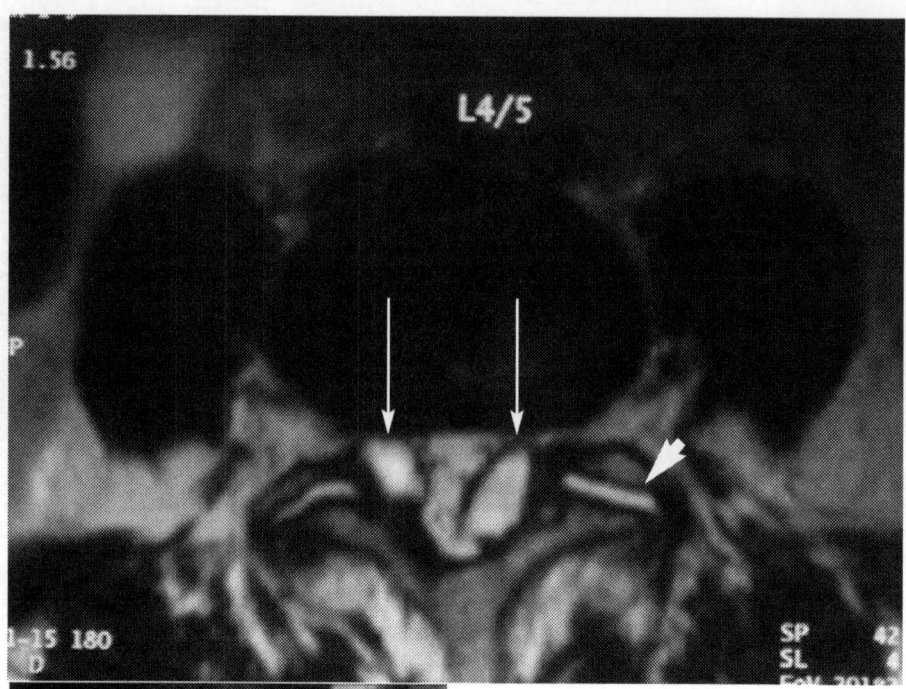

Figure 11. Synovial cysts. The image on the top is an axial T2 WI and the image on the left is a sagittal T2 WI. Note how the cysts are hyperintense and appear to arise from the facet joint (arrowhead).

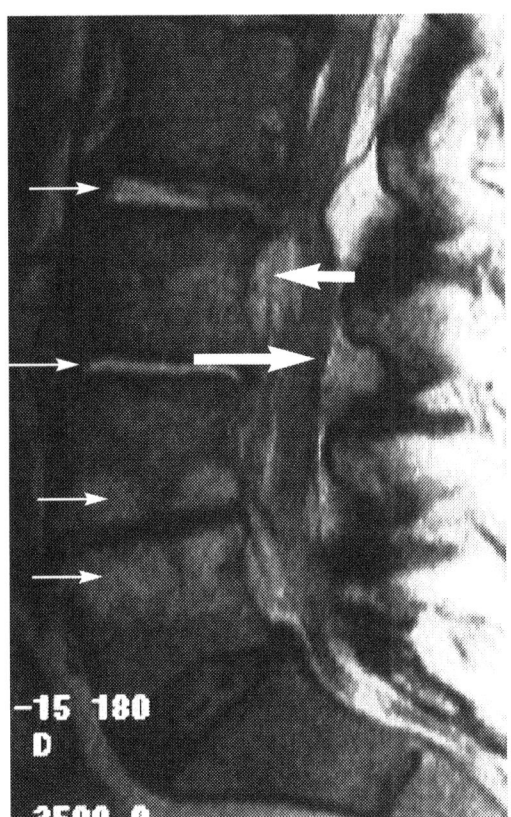

Figure 12. *This is a sagittal T2 WI of the lumbosacral spine. The two thick arrows demonstrate collections of pus, one anterior and one posterior of the cauda equina. The two top thin arrows demonstrate discitis with increased signal intensity. This is due to oedema associated with the infection of these disc spaces. The two bottom arrows demonstrate increased signal intensity in the vertebrae adjacent to the disc space signalling osteomyelitis.*

5
HEADACHE

Contents

Subarachnoid haemorrhage
Migraine
Cluster headaches
Tension headaches
Cervicogenic headaches
Headache secondary to sinusitis

There are many causes of headache and it can be quite confusing to try and decide which kind of headache is present in your patient.

Subarachnoid haemorrhage

The most relevant headache not to be missed. The sudden onset of a headache more severe than any the person has experienced before is the hallmark. It is frequently accompanied by neck stiffness, photophobia and nausea and vomiting. This is a dire emergency and immediate referral is mandated to a neurosurgeon.

Migraine

These are headaches that may have a familial connotation and usually arise early in life. It is a severe, unilateral and throbbing pain that is more common in females. Visual symptoms and associated nausea and vomiting is very common. These headaches can last for several hours and are incapacitating.

Cluster headaches

These are also severe, unilateral and usually retro-orbital with associated ocular symptoms of lacrimation and swelling of the eye. There is a male preponderance, they occur at night and tend to last for less than an hour. They may recur during the day in several separate attacks. The typical feature is that the patient will have a period of several months without symptoms.

Tension headaches

There is an associated stressor or depression present. The headaches are bilateral and frequently suboccipital and are throbbing in nature. They are more typical later in the day and tend not to be as severe in the mornings. There is no familial connotation. Associated nausea, visual or ocular symptoms are unusual. These headaches tend to last for hours to days.

Cervicogenic headaches

The fifth cranial nerves spinal nucleus descends to the mid cervical spine. Compression of the spinal cord at that level can lead to severe, usually unilateral, occipital headaches that spread frontally and typically refers to an eye. These headaches can also be caused secondary to facet joint pathology which causes cervical muscle spasm and subsequent occipital headaches.

Headache secondary to sinusitis

It is common to have localised tenderness over the sinuses. Associated nausea, visual or ocular symptoms are unusual. Infective or allergic sinusitis is frequently present. Associated nasal obstruction is also frequently present. Headaches can be chronic and last as long as the sinusitis is present.

6

BRAIN TUMOURS

Contents

Epidemiology
Genetics factors in brain tumours
Environmental factors in brain tumours
Neuropathology
Tumours according to anatomical distribution
Tumours according to classification
Pathophysiology
Clinical presentation
Investigations
Management
Prognosis

Epidemiology

The annual incidence of primary brain tumours is about 10-20 per 100,000 person years. Brain tumours are either primary or secondary. Primary brain tumours can be divided according to their histology. The most prevalent primary brain tumours are meningiomas which occur in about 25% of all primary brain tumours, followed by glioblastomas which occur in about 23%. Astrocytomas occur in around 11% and nerve sheath tumours follow at 8%. Ependymomas, oligodendrogliomas, medulloblastomas, craniopharyngiomas, pituitary tumours and lymphomas all individually constitute less than 5% each of all primary brain tumours.

Genetic factors in brain tumours

Brain tumours are caused by a combination of unchecked proliferation of a cell line as well as decreased apoptosis. This occurs when there is loss of control of the cell cycle and of programmed cell death (apoptosis). The cell cycle and cell death are normally well controlled and is disrupted by a combination of a suppression or inactivation of tumour suppression genes and an over expression and amplification of oncogenes. This occurs due to the accumulation of a series of genetic mutations.

Tumour suppressor genes - In brain tumours, the most frequently found genetic aberration is that of the tumour suppressor gene *p53* located on chromosome 17p. The *p53* gene is a transcription factor that induces and suppresses several genes that have influences on the cell cycle, genomic stability and programmed cell death. This mutation of the *p53* gene happens early in the series of genetic alterations that occur and is present in more than 50% of all gliomas. The *p53* protein up regulates the transcription of the *p21* gene that blocks the cell in the G_1 phase. Another effect of the *p53* protein is to up regulate BAX (BAX proteins regulate apoptosis in cellular pathways), which promotes apoptosis. The absence of this protein (and resultant decrease in *p21* and BAX) leads to uncontrolled cell proliferation. Other important suppressor genes are located on chromosome 9p (gene *16p*), chromosome 22q and chromosome 10.

Oncogenes – Gene amplification is a common activation pathway for oncogenes which leads to an overstimulation of growth. There are three sets of growth factors implicated in the formation of glial tumours. These growth factors all have tyrosine receptors and are epidermal growth factor (chromosome 7), platelet derived growth factor (chromosome 17p) and basic fibroblast growth factor. Another group of oncogenes on chromosome 12q inactivate the gene products of tumour suppression genes.

Environmental factors in brain tumours

There are several risk factors that may play a role such as exposure to ionising radiation, non-ionising radiation (electro magnetic field radiation), maternal alcohol consumption, chronic aspartame ingestion, exposure to vinyl chloride, infections like tuberculosis and HIV and previous cranial trauma.

Neuropathology

Most histological specimens are interpreted with hematoxylin and eosin staining. There are other stains to assist the pathologist in differentiating tissues. Reticulin is useful in differentiating meningiomas and pericytomas, and trichrome is useful in differentiating collagen and glial tissue.

Immunohistochemistry is probably the most useful adjunct in neuropathology:

Glial fibrillary acidic protein (GFAP) is a filamentous protein that is specifically expressed by astrocytes and therefore astrocytic tumours or tumours that are mixed and contain astrocytes express it. Up to 50% of ependymomas also express it.
Neuron specific enolase (NSE), synaptophysin and neurofilament, as their names suggest, are expressed by neuronal tumours as well as medulloblastomas.
Meningiomas and choroid plexus tumours express *epithelial membrane antigen (EMA)*.
Leucocyte common antigen as well as B and T-cell markers are expressed by lymphomas.

Markers of cell proliferation help to build up a biological profile of a tumour. Bromodeoxyuridine, Ki-67 and MIB-1 are markers that are frequently used. Bromodeoxyuridine is a thymidine analogue that is taken up by cells in the S-phase of the cell cycle and Ki-67 and MIB-1 is expressed by cells in all phases of the cell cycle except for G_0

Tumours according to anatomical distribution
Tumours of the skull base
Skull base tumours are difficult to treat since they abut critical neurological and vascular structures and complete resection is difficult if not impossible. A clue to the possible diagnosis might be gained from the anatomical location of the tumour. The anterior cranial fossa contains meningiomas, esthesioneuroblastomas and sometimes nasopharyngeal carcinomas; the posterior cranial fossa contains tumours of the CPA and on the floor of the posterior cra-

nial base; chordomas, chondrosarcomas and paragangliomas. The middle cranial fossa may contain chordomas, craniopharyngiomas, pituitary adenomas, metastases and meningiomas.

Suprasellar tumours
This area may contain arachnoid cysts, Rathke's cleft cysts, pituitary adenomas, craniopharyngiomas, giant aneurysms, meningiomas and metastases. Approaches are transsphenoidal and transcranially. Transcranial approaches are via subfrontal or pterional approaches.

Tumours of the CPA (cerebellopontine angle)
This area may contain epidermoid cysts, dermoid cysts, arachnoid cysts, choroid plexus tumours, schwannomas, metastases and meningiomas. Access to it is via a retromastoid, middle fossa or translabyrinthine approach.

Tumours of the posterior fossa
Posterior fossa astrocytomas are no different in character to the supratentorial variant. The main differential diagnosis for a tumour in the posterior fossa in children is that of medulloblastoma, ependymoma and astrocytoma. Medulloblastomas usually are in the midline with astrocytomas and ependymomas being off-centre. Astrocytomas (especially pilocytic astrocytomas) are more frequently cystic than ependymomas.

Intraventricular tumours
These can be ependymomas, subependymomas, choroid plexus tumours, meningiomas, subependymal giant cell astrocytomas or central neurocytomas.

Pineal region tumours
These tumours most commonly cause obstructive hydrocephalus, Parinaud's syndrome (paresis of upward gaze) and nystagmus. The differential diagnosis for tumours in this region include germ cell tumours, pineal parenchymal tumours, pineal cysts, meningiomas, dermoids and epidermoids, gliomas and vascular abnormalities like aneurysms.

Tumours according to classification

A brief classification is as follows:

Primary brain tumours

1. Neuroepithelial tissue

	Astrocytes	Astrocytoma
	Oligodendrocytes	Oligodendroglioma
	Ependyma	Ependymoma
	Choroid plexus	Choroid plexus papilloma
	Pineal gland	Pineocytoma, Pineoblastoma
	Neuronal tissue	Gangliocytoma, ganglioglioma, neuroblastoma.
	Empbryonic tissue	Glioblastoma, medulloblastoma
2	Nerve sheath cells	
		Neurilemmoma, neurofibroma
3.	Meninges	Meningioma, melanoma
4.	Blood vessels	Haemangioblastoma
5.	Lymphatic tissue	Lymphoma

6.	Pituitary	Pituitary tumours
7.	Developmental malformations	Dermoid cysts, craniopharyngioma

Metastatic tumours
The brain is a common organ for metastases from several organs. Most common malignant tumours metastasize into the brain via the blood stream. However, distant spread to other organs of primary brain tumours is extremely rare.

Extension from Adjacent sites - Tumours from adjacent structures in the base of skull such as carcinoma of the ethmoid sinuses, sphenoid sinuses and pharynx may grow upwards into the intracranial cavity and present with features of an intracranial tumour.

Pathophysiology

Different types of intracranial tumours have different effects on the brain. Tumours which are extra-cerebral (extra-axial) such as those arising from the pituitary gland, meninges, cranial nerves and the skull base tend to indent and displace the brain without destroying brain tissue. As such, they produce symptoms mainly as a result of neural compression. If such tumours are sufficiently large, they act as space occupying lesions leading to increased intracranial pressure. In contrast, tumours that grow within the brain parenchyma such as the neuroepithelial tumours, in addition to displacing also destroy brain tissue and produce symptoms from impaired function depending on the area involved. The also produce raised intracranial pressure (ICP) depending on the size. In addition, many brain tumours produce a reaction in the surrounding white matter leading to cerebral oedema that also contribute to the raised ICP.

Some tumours obstruct CSF pathways producing hydrocephalus that may result in raised ICP. Tumours such as those arising from the pituitary and the hypothalamus alter endocrine function leading to either hyper secretion or hypo secretion of hormones leading to different forms of endocrine disturbances.

Clinical presentation

Patients with brain tumours present with
a. Evidence of raised ICP
b. Focal neurological deficits
c. Epilepsy
d. Psychological disturbances
e. Endocrine disturbances
f. A combination of the above.
g. Rarely tumours tend to bleed and present as spontaneous intra-cerebral haematoma

Raised ICP
Tumours that are sufficiently large act as space occupying lesions and produce raised ICP. The earliest features of raised ICP are headache, nausea, vomiting and papilloedema. The headache is usually continuous and worse in the mornings and accompanied by bouts of vomiting and nausea. It is aggravated by coughing and sneezing and tends to progressively

increase in frequency and intensity as the tumour continues to enlarge. As the ICP increases, there is progressive impairment of consciousness recognized as a drop in GCS and with brain herniation, changes in vital signs and pupillary abnormalities that can eventually lead to death if untreated.

Focal neurological deficits
With neural compression and with destruction of neural tissue, function of the region involved begin to fail resulting in focal neurological deficits relevant to that area. These take the form of limb weakness, disturbances in sensation, gait, speech, and cranial nerve palsy. Focal neurological deficits provide a clinical indication of the site of the tumour.

Epilepsy
Brain tumours, especially those involving the cerebral hemispheres may cause epileptic seizures by altering the electrical activity of the surrounding brain. The seizures may be either focal or general. Epilepsy is most common in gliomas. meningiomas and metastases.

Psychological disturbances
Disturbances in behaviour may be the presenting feature in some of the brain tumours, specially those involving the frontal lobes. It is not uncommon for patients with long standing psychiatric illnesses to be subsequently diagnosed as having brain tumours.

Endocrine disturbances
Hormonal disturbances may occur due to hyper secretion of hormones by a tumour or hypo secretion due to destruction of functioning endocrine tissue by a tumour. Endocrine disturbances are common with pituitary tumours and hyper secretion may manifest as acromegaly, Cushing's syndrome, hyper prolactinaemia. Hypo secretion leads to hypo pituitarism. Pineal tumours also may cause hormonal disturbances manifesting as altered sexual function or pigmentation.

A combination of the above.
It is not uncommon for brain tumours to exhibit a combination of features listed above, depending on the site and size of the tumour. A large brain tumour may cause raised ICP and produce focal neurological deficits due to brain displacement or destruction and also lead to impaired consciousness that may manifest as abnormal behaviour.

Spontaneous intra-cerebral haematoma.
Rarely, brain tumours which are abnormally vascular may bleed spontaneously resulting in an intra cerebral haematoma or subarachnoid haemorrhage. The patient presents with a sudden event indicating a vascular pathology which on subsequent investigation proves to be haemorrhage from a tumour.

Investigations
Most brain tumours are evident with CT scanning. MRI provides more useful information regarding site, size, vascularity, relationship to surrounding structures and distribution of surrounding brain oedema and the views may be reformatted to different planes so as to assist treatment planning. Angiography is useful if high vascularity is suspected.

Management

The different modalities of treatment for brain tumours include
1. Surgical excision
2. Radiotherapy
3. Chemotherapy

Surgical excision
Excision of the tumour helps to arrive at a tissue diagnosis, restore normal ICP and relieve neural compression. The feasibility of total excision depends on the site of the tumour and its nature. Most of the benign tumours can be completely excised with minimal damage to the brain. However, malignant tumours that infiltrate the brain can only be treated with partial excision or biopsy if damage to functioning areas of the brain with consequent unacceptable neurological disability is to be avoided. Some of the benign tumours in relatively inaccessible positions are also treated with partial excision or biopsy.

Radiotherapy
External irradiation is useful in the management of some of the malignant tumours. Most malignant brain tumours carry a poor prognosis and although radiotherapy may delay recurrence of the tumour, complete cure is often not possible. Radiotherapy is also useful in preventing recurrence or controlling growth of some of the benign tumour that are treated with partial excision and complete cure could be achieved with rare tumours such as germinoma of the pineal gland. External radiation is applied to the whole brain, or focused to the area of the tumour. Stereotactic irradiation helps to focus accurately to small areas of tissue and can be achieved with a linear accelerator or with gamma rays.

Chemotherapy
Some of the malignant tumour are treated with anti mitotic agents which is usually used as adjuvent treatment to surgery and radiotherapy.

Prognosis

Benign tumours of the brain may be cured after total excision. However, there is a tendency to local recurrence in tumours such as meningiomas and pituitary adenomas. Malignant tumours tend to recur after removal despite treatment with radiotherapy and adjuvent methods. Some tumours such as glioblastomas have a very poor prognosis and most patients die within about an year or six months. However, metastases of brain tumours outside the nervous system is extremely rare.

7

DEGENERATIVE CONDITIONS

Contents

Rheumatoid Arthritis
Intervertebral disc disease
Spondylolysis and spondylolisthesis
Spinal canal stenosis

Rheumatoid Arthritis

Rheumatoid arthritis is a chronic, relapsing inflammatory arthritis. Inflammatory pannus in the synovium of the facet joints lead to destruction of cartilage, ligaments and bone. The clinical manifestations include early morning stiffness, fatigue and a myriad of extra-articular manifestations including pericarditis, myocarditis, pulmonary nodules, pleural effusions, kerato-conjunctivitis, scleritis and many others. The cervical spine is commonly involved due to the large number of synovial joints and the disease has a predilection for the craniocervical junction. Atlanto-axial subluxation is initiated by the loss of the retaining power of the transverse ligament, inflammatory changes in the joints and changes in the quality of the odontoid process (softening and osteoporosis). Softening and loss of bone in the lateral mass of the atlas leads to basilar impression (basilar invagination refers to the congenital variety and basilar impression to the acquired variety) and upward migration of the ondotoid relative to the skull base. The combination of atlanto-axial subluxation and basilar impression leads to anterior compression of the spinal cord and ventral medulla. The radiological findings include excessive mobility on dynamic imaging, evidence of pannus formation, ventral spinal cord compression and upward migration of the peg. Patients present with pain and myelopathy and in cases of compression of the medulla oblongata, present with brainstem dysfunction. Treatment is with atlanto-axial fixation. Severe cases of anterior pannus formation might require transoral resection of the pannus.

Intervertebral disc disease

The intervertebral disc is made up of a central, soft nucleus pulposus made up of a protein-polysaccharide mix and a retaining fibrous annulus fibrosus. Degeneration and trauma can lead to damage of the annulus fibrosus and herniation of the soft nuclear material into the intraspinal space.

There are 4 stages of disc herniation, see figure 1:

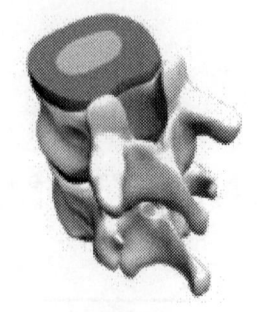

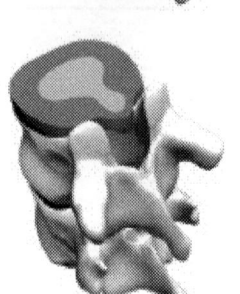

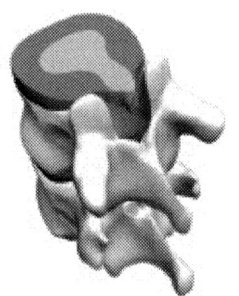

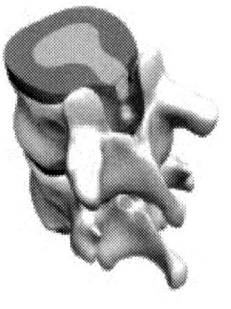

Figure 1. *Intervetebral disc herniation.*

Stage 1 (degeneration, annular tear, bulge): There are chemical changes in the disc and it appears black on T2 WI (MRI). There disc bulges but the nucleus pulposus does not breach the annulus.

Stage 2 (protrusion, prolapse): The nucleus pulposus of the disc breaks through some of the annular fibres but does not extend beyond the anatomical space usually occupied by the disc.

Stage 3 (extrusion): The nucleus pulposus of the disc breaks through the annulus and extends beyond the anatomical space usually occupied by the disc and into the spinal canal.

Stage 4 (sequestered fragment, migrated fragment, free fragment): The disc fragment breaks off and loses continuity with the rest of the disc and lies loose in the spinal canal.

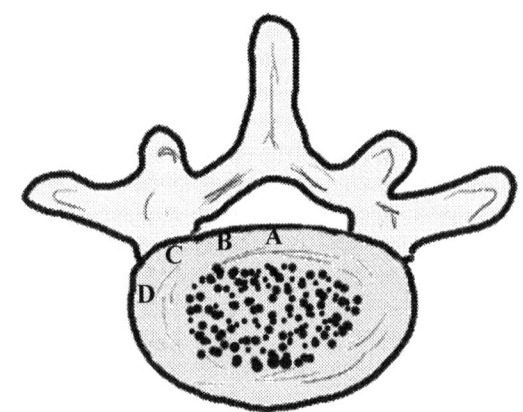

Figure 2. *The possible anatomical positions of a disc herniation is demonstrated A: Central disc herniation; B: Lateral disc herniation; C: Foraminal disc herniation and D Extraforaminal (far lateral) disc herniation.*

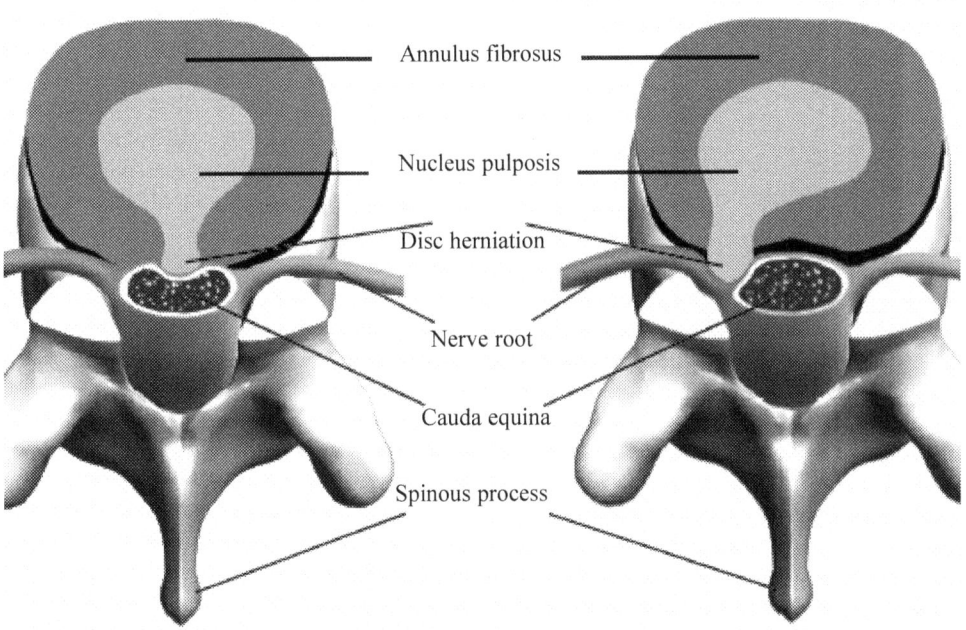

Figure 3. *The image on the left demonstrates a central disc herniation and the image on the right demonsrates a foraminal disc herniation. In these cases the herniations are in the lumbar spine and the effect of the foraminal herniation is that of a radiculopathy and in the central herniation it may be that of a cauda equina syndrome or radiculopathy. If the herniation was in the thoracic or cervical spine, the central herniation would lead to myelopathy and the foraminal herniation to a radiculopathy.*

Depending on the size, level and whether the disc is central, lateral, foraminal or far lateral, several possible clinical syndromes can ensue. Centrally herniated discs can compromise all the nerves below the level that they are located at if they are very large. The nerve roots leave the spinal canal by curling around and beneath the pedicle of the same named level in the thoracic and lumbar spines. For instance, the L4 nerve root curls around the pedicle of L4 vertebra, which is quite laterally situated and just above the disc space, therefore a central and lateral disc prolapse at L4/5 will not normally affect the L4 nerve root but the nerve roots lower down. In cases where the L4/5 disc prolapse is foraminal or extraforaminal the L4 nerve root on that side will be compressed.

Patients with early stages of disc disease may present initially with lower back pain (LBP) alone and this is thought to occur because of stretching of pain fibres in the annulus fibrosus. When the nuclear material herniates through the annulus fibrosus and compresses the nerve roots, this irritation, which is thought to be both mechanical and chemical, leads to radicular signs. Radicular signs can be lancing pain, paresthesia and motor weakness. The examination of lumbar disc disease includes the findings of a positive straight- leg raising test, the presence of sensory abnormalities or motor deficits.

See the chapter on history and examination for the dermatomes and myotomes affected by each level of disc prolapse. The examination of a patient with a prolapsed cervical disc herniation relies on the same principles and depending on the area of the paresthesias, sensory deficit and motor findings; the level of the prolapse can be fairly accurately defined. Remember that in the cervical spine a named root emerges above the pedicle of the same named vertebra - for example the left C6 nerve root passes through the left C5/6 intervertebral foramen. The obvious exceptions to the rule above is the C8 nerve roots which transverse the C7/T1 foramina. The distribution of the paresthesia in the affected dermatome is frequently the best indicator for the level of the pathology. There is a definite place for conservative management of prolapsed discs as some of them will resolve spontaneously. This is because the herniated nuclear matter, which is mostly made up of water, may dehydrate and shrink.

The accepted indications for lumbar discectomy are:
Massive midline prolapses with resultant cauda equina syndrome.
Significant motor dysfunction and weakness of a specific myotome.
Radicular pain that persists despite conservative management.
Relapses of acute LBP and sciatica that prohibits a patient from having a normal lifestyle, especially if these tend to be progressive with shorter symptom-free periods.

The possible complications of lumbar disc surgery include the following:
Damage to the cauda equina and paralysis or paresis of bladder and bowel function and variable dysfunction of the motor fibres below the level of the surgery. Also CSF leaks, post operative infection including discitis, empyema and superficial infection and post operative wound haematomas. Post operative residual or recurrent disc fragments can be differentiated from scar tissue by virtue of the fact that on T1 WI (MRI) with Gadolinium contrast enhancement, the scar tissue enhances and the disc material does not. It may however be very difficult to make the diagnosis.

Indications for a cervical discectomy:
Myelopathy (spasticity secondary to cord compression)
Muscle weakness and atrophy
Progressive radicular pains
Persisting radicular pains that prohibit a patient from having a normal lifestyle.
Foraminal cervical disc herniations can in some instances also be relieved by posterior foraminotomies which are less invasive and have been performed as day cases. Possible com-

plications following anterior cervical discectomy include damage to the recurrent laryngeal nerve with resultant vocal cord dysfunction and hoarseness, CSF leak, damage to the spinal cord, damage to the trachea, oesophagus and carotid artery (or dislodging an intra-arterial cholesterol plaque), infection and wound haematoma. A complication of a left anterior approach is damage to the thoracic duct.

Spondylolysis and spondylolisthesis

Spondylolysis is a defect in the pars interarticularis between the vertebrae of the lumbar spine and this leads to a forward slip or spondylolisthesis of one vertebra on another. Severe cases of spondylolisthesis may require fusion and the decision is usually based on the demonstration of a change in the degree of slip on dynamic flexion and extension lateral spine images. There are 5 grades which are based on the percentage of slippage of the superior vertebral body in relation to the inferior vertebral body:
Grade 1: 25%
Grade 2: 25-50%
Grade 3: 50-75%
Grade 4: 75-100%
Grade 5: greater than 100%

There are several types of spondylolisthesis:
Type 1 - Congenital: Facet dysplasia and abnormal orientation of the facet with secondary elongation of the pars interarticularis is the hallmark of this type and age of onset is usually before the age of 20.
Type 2 - Isthmic: A stress fracture of the pars interartricularis is responsible for this type. There is an association with contact sports and with the congenital type due to the biomechanical stresses placed on the pars by the orientation of the facet joints.
Type 3 - Degenerative: This is spondylolisthesis without a pars defect and is secondary to hyper mobility of the facet joints and disc pathology and results in lateral recess stenosis. Following decompression a decision to fuse should be made on a case for case basis.
Type 4 -Traumatic: Severe traumatic forces, especially hyper flexion forces can lead to fractures of the pars interarticularis.
Type 5 - Pathological: This is associated with pathological fractures of the pars.
Type 6 - Post surgical: Laminectomy carries the definite risk of spondylolisthesis and some surgeons try and limit the extent of their surgical procedures as much as possible for this reason. Posterior instrumentation subjects adjacent motion segments to endure added biomechanical stresses and the development of para fusion-segment spondylolisthesis is well known.

Spinal canal stenosis
Cervical stenosis
Spinal stenosis is either congenital or acquired and is narrowing of the spinal canal diameter due to several factors. Congenitally narrow canals and cases of acquired stenosis with canal diameters of less than 14mm are a risk factor for developing cord compression and myelopathy. The purest form of congenital spinal stenosis occurs in achondroplasia. This condition is characterised by increased periosteal bone formation and patients have abnormal vertebrae with trapezoidal shapes, shortened and thick pedicles and hypertrophied laminae. Acquired spinal stenosis can be caused by anterior compression from herniated discs, osteophytic bars, ossification of the posterior longitudinal ligament, subluxation of the vertebrae and vertebral

compression fractures. Posterior and lateral compression may be caused by hypertrophy of the ligamentum flavum and the facet joints.

The clinical syndrome depends whether there is purely radicular compromise with lateral recess and neural foramina stenosis which produces a radiculopathy (pain, paresthesia, lower motor neurone motor weakness and decreased reflexes) or whether there is compression of the cord with resultant myelopathy (spasticity, upper motor neurone weakness). Myelopathic patients have a spastic quadriparesis and problems with fine motor control of the upper limbs and a spastic gait. These patients may present with a central cord syndrome where they have greater impairment of their arm function than their leg function if they suffer a hyperextension injury. This is because of the critical narrowing of the spinal canal which leads to the spinal cord being contused in such a fall, with damage to the central cord (see chapter 12). Treatment is by decompression and the approach is dictated by the pathology with the rule generally being that anterior compression needs anterior surgery and posterior compression, posterior surgery. Anterior surgery includes anterior cervical discectomy and vertebral corpectomy and posterior surgery would include laminectomy, laminotomy and foraminotomy.

Lumbar spinal canal stenosis

This is characterised by a clinical syndrome of radicular complaints, neurogenic (spinal) claudication and symptoms of cauda equina compression secondary to direct mechanical compression and indirect vascular insufficiency. Patients with lumbar spinal canal stenosis report reduced walking distances and decreased ability to stand for long periods. The spinal claudication is typically an aching pain in their calves that is reduced with rest but even more so with a change in posture and patients will report that sitting down or squatting is helpful. The condition is manifested by a decreased canal diameter on imaging with associated facet joint hypertrophy and ligamentum flavum hypertrophy. Treatment for this condition is spinal decompression with generous fenestrations (laminotomies) or laminectomy without or with fusion. The decision on fusion is based on demonstrating instability (movement) on flexion and extension images.

8

HYDROCEPHALUS

Contents

Hydrocephalus
Childhood hydrocephalus
Adult hydrocephalus
Normal pressure hydrocephalus
Benign intracranial hypertension (pseudotumour cerebri/ idiopathic intracranial hypertension)
Shunt complications

Hydrocephalus

CSF is produced in the brain through an active process by the choroid plexus and ependyma and is passively reabsorbed by the arachnoid villi. An adult produces about 20mls of CSF every hour (0.5L per day) and the adult ventricular system contains approximately 150mls CSF. There is a very fine balance between production and absorption of CSF and, with the large volume of CSF produced every day, obstruction in the pathway of CSF flow or decreased reabsorption will lead to a build up of fluid and increase in the size of the ventricles (ventriculomegaly). Ventriculomegaly is called hydrocephalus if the ventricles are enlarged because of fluid build up. In older people, the reduced size of the brain might lead to the ventricular spaces and subarachnoid spaces enlarging due to shrinkage of the brain, and this is not called hydrocephalus but purely brain atrophy with secondary ventriculomegaly (hydrocephalus ex vacuo).

Childhood hydrocephalus

This can be either congenital or acquired. A large proportion of childhood hydrocephalus is congenital and nearly half of those cases are due to aqueduct stenosis of which there are several anatomical variants which include small multi-channels and membranes across the lumen of the aqueduct. These children frequently become hydrocephalic in utero and this can be diagnosed in perinatal ultrasonic screening. Another cause of congenital childhood hydrocephalus is Chiari malformations. Chiari 2 malformation found in children is frequently associated with myelomeningocele. Up to 90% of patients with myelomeningocele will have associated Chiari 2 malformations and up to 80% of these children will also have associated hydrocephalus. This is particularly true for lesions higher up in the spinal cord. Chiari 2 malformation consists of downwards displacement of the vermis of the cerebellum and the fourth ventricle into the cervical spinal canal. The displaced tissue is fused to the underlying brain stem and this causes hydrocephalus by blocking the foramen of Magendie. These children need combination therapy of closure of the myelomeningocele and VP shunting.

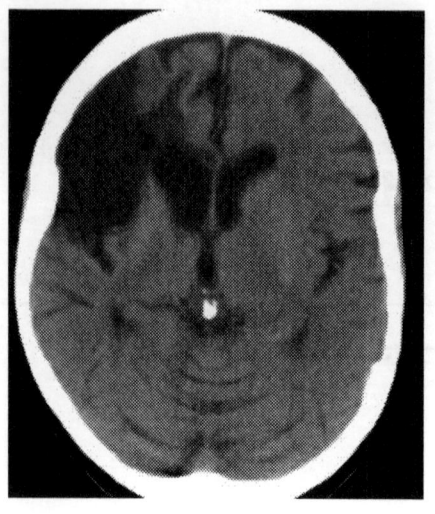 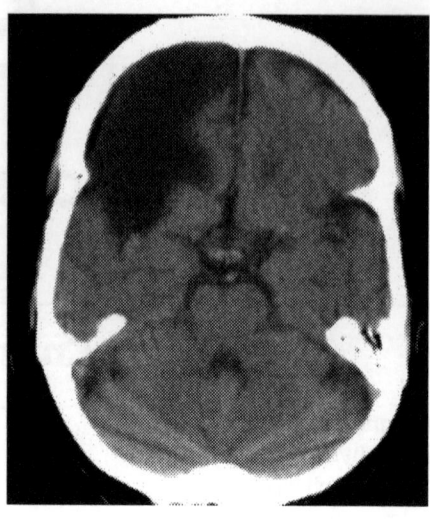

Figure 4. *Porencephalic cyst. These images are axial T1 WI and demonstrates a porencephalic cyst. A porencephalic cyst is a cavity within the cerebral hemisphere, filled with cerebrospinal fluid, that communicates directly with the ventricular system. The image on the right demonstrates the communication with the ventricle.*

Cysts are other causes of congenital hydrocephalus. Porencephalic cysts (cysts within the brain parenchyma), arachnoid cysts (cysts within the subarachnoid space) and Dandy-Walker cysts can cause hydrocephalus by compression of the ventricular system or of its outlet foramina. A Dandy-Walker cyst is a posterior fossa cyst that is in communication with the enlarged fourth ventricle with associated aplasia of the vermis of the cerebellum.
This has to be distinguished from a mega cisterna magna (large cisterna magna without hypoplasia of the vermis). Hydrocephalus is caused due to atresia of the foramina of Magendie and hydrocephalus with associated Dandy-Walker cyst is seen. The main differential diagnosis of a Dandy-Walker cyst is an arachnoid cyst of the posterior fossa and a mega cisterna magna. Another congenital form of hydrocephalus is caused by aneurysms of the vein of Galen that causes obstruction of the CSF pathway.

Acquired hydrocephalus can be obstructive due to childhood tumours or can be communicating due to post-inflammatory hydrocephalus and obstruction of the basal cisterns. Tuberculous meningitis, *Escherichia Coli* meningitis and *Haemophilus Influenza* meningitis are all well known to cause this. Premature infants weighing less than 0.5kg at birth, frequently develop intraventricular haemorrhage which can lead to obstruction of the CSF pathways. The incidence of these bleeds can be reduced with phenobarbital. Repeated CSF tapping and treatment with Diamox (acetazolamide), which reduces the production of CSF, can frequently treat communicating hydrocephalus. Persistent cases, however, need shunting. Patients with obstructive hydrocephalus may be treated by removal of the obstruction and opening of the CSF pathways but in some cases temporary CSF diversion with ventriculostomy is required or permanent diversion with third ventriculostomy or ventriculoperitoneal shunting (VPS).

Adult hydrocephalus

In adults, obstructive hydrocephalus, which is characterised by dilatation of only a part of the ventricular system, is caused by external compression of the ventricular system as in aqueduct stenosis or intraventricular obstruction by masses or bleeds. Obstructive hydrocephalus is usually treated by ventriculoperitoneal shunting. Obstructive hydrocephalus caused by aqueduct stenosis, either congenital or due to external compression, can also be treated by endoscopic third ventriculostomy. Communicating hydrocephalus (non obstructive) is due to dysfunctional absorption of CSF.

Normal pressure hydrocephalus (NPH) is a condition that occurs mostly in people older than 60. NPH is a misnomer however since it has been found that in these individuals the intracranial pressures, although mostly normal, are periodically transiently high. The condition is characterised by enlarged ventricles on imaging and a clinical triad of dementia, ataxia and incontinence. This supports dysfunction in the region of the medial frontal lobes. In about half the patients with NPH, there is a defined cause such as trauma, meningitis or subarachnoid haemorrhage which can be held accountable for the reduced absorption of CSF. The mechanism is thought to be blockage of the subarachnoid fluid pathways and blockage of some of the arachnoid villi which reabsorb CSF passively. The term idiopathic NPH is reserved for cases where there is no known cause for the hydrocephalus. Investigating NPH includes monitoring the intracranial pressure with pressure monitors, measuring the CSF pressure with a lumbar puncture (patient in decubitus position), infusing CSF through a lumbar puncture whilst measuring intracranial pressure and therapeutic drainage of CSF through either a lumbar puncture or an indwelling lumbar drain and measuring improvement in walking and mental function by the neuropsychologist. Treatment is with permanent CSF diversion via either a Lumboperitoneal or VP shunt.

Benign intracranial hypertension (BIH) also called pseudotumour cerebri or idiopathic intracranial hypertension is a disorder of unknown aetiology which affects predominantly obese women of childbearing age. The condition is characterised by raised intracranial pressure, headaches and visual disturbances secondary to papilloedema and optic nerve damage. There is thought to be either abnormalities of the arachnoid granulations or some form of venous outflow obstruction that accounts for the condition. On imaging the ventricles are usually slit-like and compressed by a generally 'tight' and swollen brain. The management is based on careful ophthalmological follow up since blindness is the major complication of this condition. Medical treatment is based on weight loss, diuretic treatment and acetazolamide (Diamox) administration. Diamox is a carbonic anhydrase inhibitor and decreases CSF production. When medical therapy fails optic nerve fenestrations are an option as well as CSF diversion with lumboperitoneal shunting. Some surgeons employ subtemporal decompression.

Shunt complications

Presentation
Beyond the age of 2 years shunt underdrainage presents with signs and symptoms of raised intracranial pressure. Up to the age of 2 years, the pliant skull and open cranial sutures allow for some compensation and resultant macrocephaly. Headaches that are worse in the recumbent position, nausea, vomiting and photophobia are typical symptoms. Patients that are completely shunt dependant and have complete occlusions typically become unwell very quickly. Considering that we produce nearly 500ml of CSF every day, this is not entirely surprising.

About 50% of shunt complications are due to malfunction of the shunt unit, approximately 20% are due to symptoms related to pressure changes or overdrainage and about 10% are due to infection.

Infection
An infection rate of 5 – 10% is the accepted norm. Most infections are usually diagnosed within two months. *Staphylococcus Epidermidis* (40%) and *Staphylococcus Aureus* (20%) are the most frequently diagnosed organisms. Most of these infections have their origin in the perioperative period. Late infections after 2 months are usually due to bowel organisms (Gram negative Bacilli). Immediately after shunt placement a glycoprotein layer forms over the shunt. There are receptors on this glycoprotein layer that present for bacterial adhesion, but if normal body cells bind on these before bacteria can, this gives a barrier against infection. It is during this period of adhesion that a sterile enviroment needs to be insured. If there is bacterial adhesion, then bacterial multiplication follows with formation of a biofilm containing bacteria, polymers and caught up cells. Clinical infection is the last stage. The biofilm gives very good protection against anti bacterial agents such as antibiotics, white cells, surfactants and antibodies. *Staphylococcus Epidermidis* is much better at producing a biofilm than *Staphylococcus Aureus*. There are three main ways that the shunt can become colonised: the first is primary colonisation at the time of surgery, the second mechanism is haematogenous spread of infection and the third is transmission of an intra-abdominal infection.

The clinical effects of infection can be local infection around the shunt, meningitis, peritonitis, obstruction or cor pulmonale and nephritis in the case of ventriculoatrial shunts. Useful adjuncts in making the diagnosis are a blood white cell count, C-reactive protein, erythrocyte sedimentation rate and blood cultures. CSF sampling is 95% accurate and can be done from the shunt reservoir or LP. A CT scan is mandatory for comparison of ventricular size.

Risks for shunt infection are young patient age, poor skin condition, concomitant systemic infections at the time of shunt placement, postoperative wound dehiscence, prolonged operation time, limited surgeon experience, shunt revision rather than primary procedure, surgery done after hours, cases where the indication for shunt placement is myelomeningocele and importantly, an increased number of people in the operating room.
Some units have reported shunt infection rates of less than 2% by aggressively focusing on these factors and trying to eliminate them.
Management of the infected shunt is aimed at maintaining continued CSF drainage and eradication of the infection. In managing an infected shunt there are basically three options. The first and least successful option is to leave the shunt in position and to administer IV antibiotics. The second option is to externalise the distal end of the shunt, administer IV antibiotics

and, if the CSF obtained from the distal end is clear, then to replace the shunt. The third option is to completely remove the shunt and place an external ventricular drain, monitor the CSF drainage and, as soon as this is clear following antibiotic treatment, replace the whole shunt. The last option is the most successful and should be the aim in all cases. It is usual practice to give prophylactic antibiotics at the time of shunt placement and there is good evidence for this in the literature.

Mechanichal failure

In 20- 40% failures present within one year. After one year the incidence is 5% per year. The mean time until revision for a standard valve is 5 yrs. It is imperative that all valves are tested at surgery for failure.

Occlusions - cause up to 50% of shunt dysfunction in pediatric population. The risk is highest immediately post operatively secondary to debris or improper ventricular catheter placement Late occlusions can be due to choroid plexus, ependymal reactions or immune reactions. Ventricular catheter occlusion can be due to debris in the CSF, improper location of the ventricular catheter point and slit ventricles (up to 40% incidence of proximal obstruction). Valve occlusions can be due to a factory fault, accumulation of debris with insertion, bacterial proliferation or immune reaction. There may be relative obstruction to flow from ascites or a pseudocyst in a ventriculo peritoneal shunt or thrombi in the lumen of a ventriculoatrial shunt. Suggestions to reduce occlusions are to make sure that the shunt inserted is clean, to place the ventricular catheter in area of most ventricular dilatation, to check patency of the valve before insertion and to choose the appropriate shunt and shunt setting to avoid over drainage and slit ventricles.

Disconnection or fracture - this is the second most frequent reason for dysfunction in the pediatric population. Reasons are improper selection of shunts, loose ties, the use of absorbable sutures, multiple connections and a rough technique during insertion.

Migration - very low profile and streamlined valves and reservoirs may be prone to migration and occlusion. Improper fixation of the shunt and excess tubing is another reason for migration and subsequent kinking and occlusion.

Improper placement of the ventricular catheter - usually directly related to the surgeon's experience.

Skin complications and subcutaneous CSF accumulations

Skin complications are seen in patients with open wounds, septic and potentially septic areas adjacent to the shunt or its tract. Poor host immune system, poor placement of the valve and large valves with sharp edges are also potentially dangerous. CSF fluid collections are seen when shunt is non functioning or when functioning but under the following conditions: loose skin, valves with high pressure, large ventricles with relatively small area of cortex or large dural openings

Overdrainage

Overdrainage occurs in up to 10% of children and 30% of adults. A standard low resistance, medium pressure valve can allow drainage of 200ml/hr in a 25cm water differential pressure. The production of CSF is only 21ml/hr. There are large variations in pressure gradients during different physiological conditions such as postural changes, REM sleep and physical exertion. The risk of overdrainage can be decreased by: increasing the opening pressure of the valve, adding an anti siphoning device or adding a flow regulatory device. The complications of overdrainage are subdural fluid collections, slit ventricles, craniostenosis, loculation of ventricles and orthostatic hypotension

9

CEREBRAL INFARCTION AND HAEMORRHAGE

Contents

Cerebral haemorrhage
Cerebral infarction

Cerebral infarction and haemorrhage are common cerebro-vascular accidents which present as a sudden onset of a neurological deficit with or without loss of consciousness. Loss of consciousness is more common with cerebral haemorrhage than with infarction.

Cerebral haemorrhage

Spontaneous haemorrhage into the brain parenchyma (intra cerebral haemorrhage or ICH) occurs when a blood vessel usually under arterial pressure ruptures into the brain substance. This could occur due a variety of reasons which are similar to those causing spontaneous sub-arachnoid haemorrhage (SAH). Indeed, it is not uncommon for spontaneous SAH to co-exist with ICH.

Pathophysiology
When a blood vessel under arterial pressure ruptures into the brain substance, the strong jet of blood cuts through the soft brain with an acute increase in intracranial pressure. This acute rise in ICP could result in immediate loss of consciousness. The point of rupture is usually sealed with a thrombus and the extravasated blood collects in a pool within the brain parenchyma. The pool of blood soon coagulates to form a solid blood clot.
The subsequent clinical picture depends on the size of the blood clot and the location. If the blood clot is relatively small, there could be sufficient compensation within the intracranial cavity so that any mass effect is minimal. However, if the clot is of a sufficiently large size, it acts as a space occupying lesion and causes increased ICP and brain displacement. Raised ICP could also be caused by an ICH blocking CSF pathways such in the cerebellum resulting in obstructive hydrocephalus.
Following the initial haematoma formation, there is commonly secondary change in the damaged brain parenchyma due to various chemicals that are released in the region of the ICH. These result in a degree of cerebral oedema that would further contribute to the raised ICP and also extend the area of brain damage beyond the confines of the original ICH.
Depending on the location of the clot, there could be focal neurological deficits. The dam-

age done to the brain when the jet of blood cuts through would result in disruption of white matter pathways leading to loss of function in the relevant areas. The common deficits are hemiparesis, cerebellar signs and multiple cranial nerve palsy in case of brain stem ICH. If the ICH occupies a 'silent' area of the brain, there would be no focal neurological deficit.

Clinical features
Patients with spontaneous ICH present with a sudden onset of a neurological deficit with or without loss of consciousness. There is frequently accompanying headache. Changes in GCS score, size of the pupils and vital signs may be present depending on the extent of raised ICP caused by the ICH. CT scans show the site and extent of the ICH as well as complications such as hydrocephalus or accompanying oedema.

Management
The management is directed towards identifying a cause for the haemorrhage and treating the ICH.
Identification of the cause of the haemorrhage involves estimation INR and investigation of other clotting abnormalities as well identifying systemic hypertension and appropriate management. In the absence of a systemic cause, angiography is used to identify any local abnormality of blood vessels.
If the ICH is of a sufficiently large size and causing raised intra-cranial pressure, it has to be evacuated as an emergency to prevent irreversible brain damage due to uncontrolled ICP. If the ICH is relatively small, it would re-absorb with time and treatment is directed towards the cause of the haemorrhage and prevention of future recurrence depending on the cause. This is achieved by surgical, endovascular or radiosurgical means or a combination of these modalities.

Cerebral infarction

Cerebral infarction occurs when a blood vessel to a certain part of the brain is blocked.

Pathophysiology
Blood vessels in the brain could be blocked as a result of local thrombus formation on an atheromatous plaque or due to an embolus of distant origin. Blocking of a blood vessel proximal to the circle of Willis could be compensated to some extent depending on the integrity of the circle but the vessels beyond have minimal cross anastomoses and behave as end vessels. Obstruction to such an artery results in ischaemia in the area of supply of that artery which could lead to infarction.
There is a physiological reserve in the requirements of perfusion of brain tissue and certain degrees of cerebral ischaemia could be compensated without any evidence of cerebral dysfunction. However, when perfusion drops below the limits of this reserve, that area of brain tissue loses its function and leads to a focal neurological deficit. There is again a range in perfusion where brain tissue could lose function but not necessary undergo necrosis. Thus it is possible for the impaired cerebral function to recover following restoration of perfusion if the area involved has not undergone necrosis and irreversible infarction.
If brain tissue undergoes necrosis and infarction, there is release of chemicals to the surrounding parenchyma resulting in oedema of the white matter that could cause raised ICP and brain displacement. This process could extend the area of brain damage resulting in secondary extension of the infarct. Sometimes, extravasation of blood takes place in the infarcted brain resulting in a haemorrhagic infarct that could further extend the area of brain damage

and also further increase ICP. If the infarct and oedema involves the cerebellum, there could be obstruction to CSF pathways resulting in hydrocephalus and raised ICP.

Clinical features
Patients present with a sudden onset of a neurological deficit depending on the area of brain involved. If there is extension of the infarct and brain oedema, they may have raised ICP with impaired consciousness. The location and extent of the infarct is evident on CT scans.

Management
The management of cerebral ischaemia is mainly medical with an attempt to reduce secondary extension of the zone of ischaemia, prevention of further ischaemic episodes and rehabilitation to facilitate recovery from neurological disability.

Surgical interference is indicated in the event of complication such as obstructive hydrocephalus, and heamorrhagic infarction that may sometimes require evacuation to control raised ICP. In case of cerebellar infarction, the swelling of the cerebellum in the restricted confines of the posterior cranial fossa could lead to brain stem compression and respiratory and cardiac dysfunction. In such cases, excision of the infarcted cerebellar tissue helps to control swelling and brain stem compression.

Surgical methods are also employed for revascularisation procedures but more recently endovascular techniques such as angio-plasty are used with increasing frequency.

10
CRANIOSPINAL INFECTION

Contents

Cranial infection

Extra-axial infection
Osteomyelitis
Epidural abscess (empyema)

Intra-axial infection
Bacterial meningitis
Subdural empyema
Cerebritis and brain abscess
Ventriculitis
Viral infections
Parasitic diseases

Spinal infection
Osteomyelitis
Epidural empyema (abscess)
Subdural abscess (empyema)
Intramedullary abscess
Discitis
Tuberculosis of the spine

Cranial infection
Extra-axial infection
This includes infection of the scalp, the skull (osteomyelitis) and the epidural (extradural) compartment.
Osteomyelitis
Osteomyelitis is relatively rare and usually follows either penetrating trauma or neurosurgical intervention but may also be spontaneous. *Staphylococcus Aureus* most commonly causes the infection and the treatment includes complete debridement and long-term antibiotic cover.
Epidural abscess (empyema)
Epidural and subdural empyema have the same pathogenesis. The most common causes are penetrating trauma, neurosurgical procedures and infection of nearby anatomical spaces

(facial air sinuses, the mastoid and middle ear sinuses) and haematogenous spread is less likely. Epidural empyema is usually associated with osteomyelitis and the main complications of epidural abscess are thrombosis of nearby vascular structures and intracranial spread. In extradural empyema without any subdural spread, CSF studies are usually normal. The peripheral white blood cell count and inflammatory markers are usually elevated and the patient might be pyrexial with signs of increased intracranial pressure. Management is complete surgical evacuation and long-term antibiotic cover.

Intra-axial infection
Intra-axial cranial infection includes meningitis, subdural empyema, cerebritis, brain abscess and ventriculitis.

Bacterial meningitis
Meningitis is either aseptic or septic. Septic meningitis can be acute (within hours or days) or chronic (for at least 4 weeks) and can be iatrogenic or spontaneous. Clinically patients present with symptoms and signs that include the following: lethargy or confusion, fever, neck stiffness and Kernig's sign (meningeal irritation), photophobia, nausea and vomiting. CSF analysis shows increased white cells (leucocytosis). In bacterial or septic meningitis, there is a polymorphonuclear pleocytosis and in aseptic meningitis, a predominant lymphocytosis. Certain patient factors (age and immune status) and iatrogenic factors play a role in the type of organism involved (see table 1.) In septic meningitis CSF must be obtained emergently and the patient placed on a broad spectrum antibiotic regime (see table 2). There is usually a polymorphonuclear leukocytosis, low CSF glucose and, the gram stain will be positive in 80% of patients that have not had any antibiotic therapy. The yield drops to 50-60% in patients who have had antibiotic treatment. Aseptic meningitis, which is much more common than septic meningitis, is frequently due to a non-bacterial infective agent and less often to partially treated septic meningitis. Basic supportive and symptomatic treatment is usually all that is required in aseptic meningitis if it is of viral origin or if the cause cannot be found. If it is due to fungal or other infection, the treatment is based on the organism isolated.

Subdural empyema
This accounts for between 5 – 25% of intracranial infections. It is associated with nearby pyogenic infections (sinusitis and mastoiditis) or overlying osteomyelitis and extradural empyema. There is a classical triad - namely sinusitis, fever and neurological deficit. When the empyema progresses it acts like an intracranial mass lesion causing raised intracranial pressure. Subdural empyema leads to an intense reaction in the underlying brain causing oedema and, in cases of cortical vessel thrombosis, to infarction. A hallmark of subdural empyema, which should raise a definite suspicion of infection, is that of seizures and thus all patients should be treated with prophylactic anticonvulsants. The microbiology of the infection is related to the source of infection and sinusitis causes empyema by anaerobic organisms and less commonly by aerobic *Streptococci and Staphylococci*. In iatrogenic infections or post-traumatic infections *Staphylococcus Aureus* is the predominant organism. In children there is a pattern of subdural empyema that follows infection with *Haemophilus Influenza* and *Streptococcus Pneumonia* meningitis. Both extradural and subdural empyema are diagnosed on CT scanning with the administration of intravenous iodine contrast which demonstrates enhancement of the collection, the overlying dura and the underlying cortex. MRI scanning, however, is much more sensitive for diagnosing empyema, especially in subtemporal collections or collections that are located on the tentorium cerebelli. Coronal cuts are especially useful. Treatment is complete surgical evacuation and long-term intravenous antibiotics. These cases should be treated as an emergency as the spread of the organism and subsequent cortical thrombosis can lead to cerebral infarction and malignant brain swelling.

Age/predisposing factors	Bacteria implicated
< 3 months	Listeria Monocytogenes Group B Streptococci Eschericia Coli Haemophilus Influenzae Streptococcus Pneumoniae Neisseria Meningitidis
3 months to 50 years	Haemophilus Influenzae Streptococcus Pneumoniae Neisseria Meningitidis
Older than 50 years or immunocompromised state	Streptococcus Pneumoniae Neisseria Meningitidis Listeria Monocytogenes Aerobic gram-negative bacilli
Iatrogenic Introduction (surgery)	Staphylococcus Aureus Coagulase-negative Staphylococci Aerobic gram-negative bacilli
Fractures extending into sinuses (base of skull)	Streptococcus Pneumoniae Haemophilus Influenzae Group A Streptococci

Table 1. *The Most Common Bacteria implicated in different age groups and different clinical scenarios.*

Age/predisposing factors	Antibiotic regime
Neonates	Ampicillin plus third generation cephalosporin
Older than 1 month	Ampicillin plus third generation cephalosporin plus vancomycin
Immunocompromised state	Ampicillin plus ceftazidime plus vancomycin
Iatrogenic Introduction (surgery) and trauma	Vancomycin plus ceftazidime

Table 2. *The suggested antibiotic regime for different age groups and different clinical scenarios.*

Cerebritis and brain abscess

Infection of the brain parenchyma leading to cerebritis and brain abscess is mostly, but not exclusively, due to pyogenic bacteria. The foci that seed the parenchyma vary and bacteria can enter the CNS via several mechanisms including spread from infection in adjacent structures such as dental infection, infection of the cranial and facial sinuses, middle ear infection and from mastoiditis. The location of the intracranial infection is usually adjacent to the extra cranial infection, giving a clue as to the cause (middle and posterior fossa in mastoiditis and anterior fossa in frontal sinusitis).

It may also occur as haematogenous spread from local (retrograde thrombophlebitis) or distant sites of infection. Another mechanism is direct innoculation at the time of surgery, penetrating trauma or base of skull fractures. In children, patent dermal tracts (lumbar lipomyelomeningocele, dermal sinus etc) are a congenital cause of CNS infection. The most common organisms are the *Streptococci and Staphylococci*. When infection has spread from nearby sinuses, gram-negative bacteria are prevalent.

There are 4 stages in the evolution of cerebritis into a brain abscess.
Early Cerebritis: In the first 5 days, there is a localised but non-capsulated area of oedema, pin point haemorrhage and small areas of necrosis.
Late Cerebritis: For the next week to two weeks, the infection attains a core of central necrosis. Neovascularity in the periphery leads to contrast enhancement.
Early capsule formation: Collagen and reticulin is laid down, the surrounding oedema starts to subside and there is early gliosis around the abscess.
Late capsule formation: This may go on for months and ends up with the capsule consisting of an outer gliotic layer, a middle collagenous layer and an inner inflammatory layer.
Patients may present with seizures or symptoms due to mass effect. Treatment is that of drainage, long term antibiotic treatment and treatment with prophylactic anticonvulsants.

Ventriculitis
Ventriculitis is infection of the CSF contained in the ventricles, and this can be due to the spread of infection in other anatomical compartments, but is mostly due to infection of ventricular shunts or external ventricular drains. In cases where intraparenchymal abscesses break through into the ventricular space by rupturing through the ependyma, there is a high associated morbidity and mortality. These cases are treated aggressively by external ventricular drainage, washout of the pus from the ventricular space and systemic antibiotics.

Viral infections
Human immunodeficiency virus infection
The spectrum of neurological disorders caused by this virus is large and is a direct effect either of the infection or because of the associated immunosuppression. The direct effects are those of meningitis, encephalopathy and myelopathy. Secondary or opportunistic infections are those of other viral infections such as progressive multifocal encephalopathy (PML), which is a result of a papovavirus infection with the JC virus and fungal infections.

JC virus (PML)
This virus infects oligodendrocytes and astrocytes and is characterised pathologically by demyelination and adjoined astrocytes with abnormal oligodendrocytes. Clinically these patients usually present with limb weakness followed by cognitive dysfunction, gait disturbance, visual loss, speech and language disorder and headache. On CT scanning patients usually have hypodense white matter lesions in the centrum semi-ovale and the cerebellum. This is a very aggressive condition and the mean survival time is reported to be 2-4 months.

Cryptococcus meningitis
This is an encapsulated fungus with yeast-like properties found mainly in dirt and bird droppings. About half of the cases of *C. Neoformans* meningitis occur in immunocompromised patients, and the rest occur in patients with normal cellular immunity. This is a chronic basilar meningitis and appears to be a result of activation of primary disease with cystic lesions, containing clusters of yeast surrounded by inflammatory and reactive gliosis, throughout the cerebral cortex. Clinical presentation includes signs of increased intracranial pressure and focal neurological signs. CSF examination shows a mononuclear pleocytosis and depressed glucose with elevated protein. The CSF streptococcal antigen and serum streptococcal anti-

gen latex agglutination tests have a high degree of sensitivity and the definitive diagnosis is made on culture of the CSF. CT scan findings are usually normal. A mortality of 30% is reported. Treatment is with systemic intravenous amphoteracin B for a minimum of 6 weeks, followed by fluconazole to prevent remission.

Toxoplasma gondii

This is a protozoal infection and is one of the most common complications associated with HIV infection. It accounts for up to half of identified neurological illnesses in patients with HIV. Approximately 25-50% of patients who are serum positive for *T Gondii* develop toxoplasma encephalopathy. *T Gondii* is an intracerebral parasite that is found in mammals, and people are usually infected by eating raw or undercooked meat that contains cysts. The house cat is the normal host of this parasite. The usual presenting neurological symptoms of patients infected with toxoplasma encephalitis are local signs superimposed on encephalopathy. The course of the illness is usually subacute, over 1-2 weeks. The lesions are usually identified as multiple ring-enhancing lesions with oedema on imaging and usually they are found in the basal ganglia. The diagnosis of *T Gondii* is not always straightforward and the CSF findings may be non-specific. It is difficult to distinguish between active and chronic toxoplasma infection with western blot methods and the only definitive means of establishing a diagnosis is a brain biopsy demonstrating tachyzoites on histological examination. These need to be excision biopsies as needle biopsies may be negative. Due to this, several authors recommend that a trial of anti-toxoplasma therapy is commenced in these patients and if therapy fails a brain biopsy is then performed. Current therapy for toxoplasma is a combination therapy with Sulfadiazine and Pyrimethamine.

Herpes viruses

These include the *Herpes Simplex virus*, the *Varicella Zoster virus*, *Epstein-Barr virus* and *Cytomegalo virus*. Human herpes viruses usually infect people early in their lives. In patients with normal immune function, they don't usually cause any complications but in immuno-compromised patients they come to the fore. The *Herpes Simplex virus type 1* is usually acquired through non-sexual activities during early childhood whereas type 2 is usually sexually transmitted. *Herpes Simplex virus type 1* encephalitis is an acute haemorrhagic necrotising encephalitis with severe morbidity. The CSF is non-specific showing a mostly mononuclear leukocytosis. The CSF may be tested for the virus specific antigens. The current management is to treat these patients empirically with Acyclovir rather than performing a brain biopsy. Therefore the treatment plan is immediate treatment with Acyclovir performing a polymerase chain reaction and, if this is negative, performing a brain biopsy. Whereas the *Herpes Simplex virus type 1* usually causes encephalitis, *Herpes Simplex type 2 viruses* usually cause meningitis and the treatment for this is Acyclovir.

Epstein-Barr virus

This is the infective agent for infectious mononucleosis and the central nervous complications of this disease are meningo-encephalitis, transverse myelitis, transcending myelitis and acute encephalitis. The outcome of Epstein-Barr virus encephalitis is usually favourable. This virus also causes Bell's palsy.

Cytomegalovirus

Cytomegalovirus is also a human herpes virus that is transmitted sexually, oral to oral or via respiratory transmission. There is both a congenital and an acquired form and treatment is with Acyclovir and Foskarnet.

Prion disease

Creutzfeld-Jacob disease

Prions are particles without nucleic acid and without detectable antigenicity but retain a clear capacity for infectivity. There are three distinct manifestations of this disease. There are sporadic cases; familial cases and cases of iatrogenic transmission. Clinical presentations include dementia and deficits of higher cortical function as well as myoclonic jerks and the disease is invariably fatal although some patients have survived as long as five years. On magnetic resonance imaging, the patient demonstrates cerebellar atrophy with increased signal intensity on T2 weighted images in the region of the basal ganglia. Diagnosis is made by brain biopsy. This is a highly infective agent and the use of disposable instruments is the only way to prevent disease transmission.

Parasitic diseases
Cysticercosis *(Taenia solium)*

This is the most common parasitic disease. It is caused by the tapeworm *T solium*. Humans are the definitive host for the parasite *T solium* with pigs being the intermediate host. Patients develop cysticercosis by ingesting fertilised eggs containing the scolex of the tapeworm carrier. These eggs are digested and embryos penetrate the blood stream and pass to the brain to form cysticerci. Cysticerci are vesicles with an invaginated scolex. Cysticercosis can have a variable presentation and may appear as cysts in the parenchyma, which can lead to seizures or encephalitis but may also present in the subarachnoid space, intraventricular space or inside the cerebellum. Spinal disease is rare but has been described. Imaging reveals variable presentations of this disease. Small granulomas and calcifications depict dead parasites. Hypodense, non-enhancing lesions represent viable cysticerci and hypodense lesions that enhance are demonstrated in the encephalitic phase and this may sometimes be combined with diffuse brain swelling. In making the diagnosis, CSF is invaluable and complement-fixation test is sensitive in 80% of cases and IGM antibody in ELISA testing has 95% specificity. The management includes medical therapy, stereotactic drainage and macroscopic, open excision. Medical management is with Albendazole. Some authors have reported a chemical meningitis and encephalitis if there is spillage of the daughter cysts during surgery and some surgeons advise using steroids to cover against this eventuality.

Echinococcosis *(Echinococcus granulosus)*

E granulosus causes hydatid disease, and humans are the intermediate host with dogs being the definitive host. Sheep and pigs are also intermediate hosts. Humans ingest the eggs along with food and liquids, and embryos freed from the eggs enter the intestinal mucosa and the vascular system. The CNS manifestation is usually that of a single large cyst in the area of the middle cerebral artery territory and the presentation is usually of a young patient presenting with symptoms and signs of increased intracranial pressure. Imaging reveals a non-enhancing, cystic lesion. Serological tests are used to diagnose the condition. At surgery, the cyst should be delivered without spillage as this could result in anaphylactic shock. Many authors report using a method of saline irrigation at the cyst-brain interface.

Granulomatous disease of the central nervous system
Mycobacterium tuberculosis

M tuberculosis is an acid fast bacillus and causes systemic infection (pulmonary, gastro intestinal tract) as well as meningitis. Infection with *M tuberculosis* is mostly a disease of the developing world. Intracranial tuberculomas form following infection in another systemic location with haematogenous spread of the organism. When a tuberculoma is formed intracranially, a thick capsule forms around it secondary to the host's main reaction and these non-caseating tuberculomas may be single or multiple. The organism frequently causes a basal arachnoiditis and meningitis (especially in the paediatric population) which can lead to communicating or non-communicating hydrocephalus. CSF analysis reveals increased protein with leukocytosis and a normal glucose. On imaging, the target sign is pathognomonic of a tuberculoma and this consists of a central calcification or nidus surrounded by a ring of enhancing material. Lesions may also be cystic. These lesions respond to chemotherapy with anti-TB drugs and it is only occasionally necessary to remove the lesions to relieve mass effect. In the case of meningitis and hydrocephalus, treatment with Diamox is used to reduce CSF production. In cases of obstructive hydrocephalus, treatment is CSF diversion with ventriculoperitoneal shunting or third ventriculostomy. These patients are frequently immuno-compromised or in a poor systemic state with poor nutrition and low body weight and have a high incidence of post procedural shunt infections.

Spinal infection
Osteomyelitis
Vertebral osteomyelitis can develop from haematogenous spread, direct involvement from adjacent infection, penetrating trauma or from iatrogenic introduction of infectious agents. The onset may be quite insidious but the presentation is usually that of increasing spinal pain, accentuated by movement and may associated with radicular signs and symptoms. On examination, the spine is usually tender to palpation. *Staphylococcus Aureus* and gram negative organisms predominate as causative organisms. Concomitant epidural abscesses lead to cord or cauda equina compression and may result in neurological compromise. Blood cultures may be positive and the ESR and CRP are usually elevated, but the white cell count may not be elevated. Radionuclide scans are very sensitive for diagnosing these infections and are positive a long time before plain films show changes. CT scanning is also very sensitive, showing hypodensity at the site of the infected discs and vertebrae as well as showing gas within the vertebrae. When healing occurs of the lesions in the chronic phase, they become denser on CT. On MRI scan there are low intensity changes on T1 WI and high intensity changes on T2 WI because of the increased water content and the lesions frequently enhance with contrast. Most cases of purely bony osteomyelitis can be treated with antibiotics, bed rest and analgesia. If the organism has not been identified with blood cultures, a CT-guided needle biopsy may be necessary. If this fails, an open surgical biopsy might be indicated and if no organism is grown then empiric antibiotics should be administered. Authors differ in opinion about the length of antibiotic therapy but it is generally accepted that at least six weeks of IV antibiotics should be given. This should be monitored by testing inflammatory markers regularly and serial scanning and there should be an improvement of both parameters. Oral antibiotics may be instituted when there is a continued downward trend in the inflammatory markers and the imaging characteristics have stabilised. Because the bone becomes weak during infection, external bracing should be used for mobilisation and, after a period of mobilisation, repeat imaging should be performed. Surgery is reserved for cases that do not respond to antibiotic therapy or where there are definite mass lesions and compromise of nervous structures. This frequently requires an anterior approach with bony grafting and fusion. Permanent morbidity is related to vascular thrombosis secondary to sepsis and to neural compromise secondary to compression.

Epidural empyema (abscess)
The mode of infection is the same as for osteomyelitis. There are several predisposing factors in both of these conditions namely diabetes mellitus, immuno-incompetence, alcoholism, malignancies and chronic systemic diseases. The signs and symptoms are very similar to those of osteomyelitis as a spinal epidural abscess is frequently an extension of the osteomyelitic disease. Back pain with focal tenderness is the hallmark and this is associated in the lumbar spine with radicular compromise and conus medullaris/cauda equina syndrome

when there is significant compromise of the theca. The presentation of epidural abscesses in the thoracic and cervical spine is different. Myelopathic signs predominates and the plain films might show some bony erosion or disc space changes, but these are rare. MRI scanning of the spine is the imaging of choice showing a hypointense lesion on T1 WI which is hyperintense on T2 WI and enhances with contrast. Radionuclide scans are extremely sensitive and are usually the first imaging modality that diagnoses these lesions. These conditions are medical emergencies due to the permanent morbidity that they cause if not aggressively treated. Morbidity is secondary to vascular thrombosis or to neural compromise by direct compression. Immediate surgical decompression with concomitant antibiotic therapy is the treatment of choice. At surgery the most usual finding is that of organised infected tissue although liquid pus might also be found. The pathogen most frequently involved is *Staphylococcus Aureus and Streptococci*. In cases where the neurological deficit is secondary to vascular thrombosis the prognosis is extremely poor.

Subdural abscess (empyema)
The same risk factors and mode of spread and dissemination for this holds true as for the two previous conditions and the clinical presentation and infecting organisms are much the same. At surgery these tend to have a less granulation tissue and a more fluid consistency. Treatment is complete evacuation and broad-spectrum antibiotics.

Intramedullary abscess
These are rare lesions but have the same aetiology, presentation and management as the previous lesions. They usually appear as hypointense lesions on T1 WI and hyperintense lesions on T2 WI and enhance strongly with contrast in the intramedullary space. Treatment is with drainage and long term IV antibiotics.

Discitis

Spontaneous discitis
Spontaneous haematogenous spread or spread from nearby infection may result in discitis, as with osteomyelitis. The blood supply of the cartilage is restricted to the periphery and it is a relatively avascular structure but this does not preclude infection from occuring in an intervertebral disc. Discitis presents in a similar fashion as osteomyelitis and also has the complication of an epidural abscess. Treatment is with broad-spectrum antibiotics, bed rest and analgesia. The diagnosis is made by demonstrating raised inflammatory markers and isolating the organism from either blood culture or a direct needle aspiration biopsy.

Iatrogenic discitis
Iatrogenic discitis following spinal surgery can either be an irritant chemical discitis or infective discitis. Patients with infective discitis tend to have a higher level of inflammatory markers. The inflammatory markers usually stay elevated for about two weeks post surgery but should return to normal thereafter in cases not complicated by infection. On imaging the infected disc appears hypointense on T1 WI and hyperintense on T2 WI, demonstrating a higher fluid content and may enhance with Gadolinium contrast administration. Treatment is bed rest and antibiotics following isolation of the organism and, in cases where there is an associated fluid collection, complete drainage of the collection producing neural compromise should be performed.

Tuberculosis of the spine
Mycobacterium Tuberculosis infection of the spine is endemic in some parts of the developing world but is now also spreading to the developed world. Infection with *M Tuberculosis* starts off in the vertebra or adjacent endplate and its hallmark is destruction of the vertebra and gibbus formation with collapse of the vertebra whilst the integrity of the disc is maintained until quite late in the disease. Spinal TB can cause the destruction of several contigu-

ous levels or can result in skip lesions and in some cases can cause epidural abscesses. The disease usually begins within the metaphyseal bone and then spreads underneath the anterior longitudinal ligament. The patient may present with the effects of pulmonary TB or with spinal pain and neurological deficit. On X-ray, vertebral involvement with erosion kyphosis with mostly involvement of the vertebrae, sparing the posterior elements, is seen. There is frequently some soft tissue involvement with calcification. CT scans are quite useful in delineating the extent of the disease and skin testing is usually positive. In the developing world the treatment of spinal TB is ambulatory chemotherapy and, in the case of severe paraparesis, bed rest and chemotherapy. The cornerstone of treatment is chemotherapy rather than surgery. Surgery is reserved for cases of severe kyphosis. Deformity following chemotherapy frequently is equal to or is better than in cases of surgery. In the developed world, the movement towards surgery is more aggressive and a combination of surgery (for gibbus formation and deformity) with chemotherapy is used. It is important to understand that the correction of deformity will deteriorate over time and therefore external bracing is important whilst the patient is ambulant. In cases where there are epidural pus collections, surgery is indicated to drain the collections. The patient should be on chemotherapy for at least 6 months.

11

VASCULAR ABNORMALITIES

Contents

Intracranial vascular abnormalities
    Arteriovenous malformations (AVM)
    Cavernous angiomas
    Venous angiomas
    Cerebral aneurysms
Spontaneous subarachnoid haemorrhage (SAH)

Intracranial vascular abnormalities

The intracranial vasculature develops pathology in several ways. There may be occlusion of arteries or venous structures or haemorrhage can occur into the parenchyma, the intraventricular system, the subdural space or subarachnoid space.

Occlusion of cerebral blood vessels is usually due to embolic phenomena and these can be secondary to atherosclerotic plaques, infected emboli or foreign material. Occlusion of the arterial side of the circulation leads to ischaemia and, if the blood flow is not restored instantly, it will lead to cell death and infarction. Occlusion of the venous part of the circulation will lead to venous hypertension, intraparenchymal bleeds and infarction. Hypertensive spontaneous intraparenchymal bleeds are secondary to the rupture of friable blood vessels. Spontaneous haemorrhages can also be secondary to vascular anomalies and/or aneurysms.

Arteriovenous malformations (AVM) are lesions in which the arterial system short-circuits directly into the venous system without the intervening capillary bed. The venous circulation is not designed to function under such high pressure and this leads to tortuous vessels and associated flow aneurysms may also develop. AVM's recruit additional blood vessels and may grow quite large. They are graded according to the Spetzler-Martin grading scale based on three factors, namely the size of the lesion, its location and the type of venous drainage. AVM's either cause effects secondarily to brain irritation (seizures) or may present with spontaneous intraparenchymal bleeds.

Cavernous angiomas (cavernomas, cavernous malformations) do not fill from the systemic circulation and do not drain via veins but rather are abnormal thin-walled vascular channels (caverns). They can present with spontaneous haemorrhage or seizures and are more prevalent in the paediatric population. Cavernous angiomas are sometimes found in the spinal cord and can cause potentially devastating neurological sequelae secondary to haemorrhage.

Size	Score	Eloquent brain	Score	Deep draining vein	Score
more than 6cm	3	Yes	1	Yes	1
3-6cm	2	No	0	No	0
less than 3cm	1				

Table 1. *The Spetzler-Martin grading scale. The size of the lesion is divided into categories of less than 3cms (1 point), 3-6cms (2 points) and greater than 6cms (3 points). If the AVM is located in an eloquent area of the brain such as the speech area, motor area, visual cortex or brain stem then another point is added. If the venous draining system is deep and if the lesion, for instance, drains directly into the vein of Galen or the straight sinus, then another point is added. The maximum score therefore is five.*

Since cavernomas do not fill or drain from the systemic circulation, they are diagnosed on MRI scanning and are non-detectable on angiography. Lesions can be watched expectantly if they are discovered incidentally. Symptomatic lesions with multiple haemorrhagic events, can be treated surgically if accessible, or with radio surgery if surgically inaccessible.

Venous angiomas are most likely to have formed during the embryonic period due to an arrest of venous development. They are composed of dilated venous channels that drain normal brain and converge into medullary veins which are enlarged and these in turn drain into normal cortical veins. They may sometimes be found in association with cavernous angiomas. The majority of these lesions are discovered incidentally and present only infrequently with haemorrhage. These lesions can be diagnosed on MRI scanning as well as angiography. On contrasted MRI scanning they form a characteristic 'caput medusa lesion' where dilated capillary veins drain centrally towards a main draining vein. They can be diagnosed on angiography when, in the venous phase, a persistent pattern of dilated medullary veins is seen that drains towards a single draining vein. They are usually managed expectantly.

Cerebral aneurysms are usually found amongst the medium sized arteries of the circle of Willis and can be fusiform dilatations or saccular berry aneurysms. Saccular aneurysms form due to weakness of the interna and media of the artery wall resulting in outpouching. These are true aneurysms. False aneurysms can be found secondary to trauma or infection and are not contained by the vessel wall but rather by the surrounding tissues. Aneurysms are thought to be flow related in their mechanism of origin and are usually found at vessel bifurcation on the side of the greatest flow.

Some inherited conditions are associated with the formation of cerebral aneurysms, including polycystic kidney disease, Ehlers-Danlos syndrome, Marfan syndrome and neurofibromatosis type 1. Aneurysms, unlike the other malformations noted above, usually present with subarachnoid haemorrhage as they are located in the subarachnoid space. The other lesions usually cause intraparenchymal haemorrhage. In cases of intraparenchymal haemorrhage, the clinical effects are due to direct destruction of brain and to secondary pressure effects of the intraparenchymal clot. In the case of aneurysms that have previously leaked, the dome of the aneurysm can become adherent to brain and subsequent bleeds can also have an intraparenchymal component. Saccular (berry) aneurysms are classified according to size into small (less than 10mm), large (more than 10mm) and giant (greater than 25mm); their location in the anterior or posterior circulation of the circle of Willis and which blood vessel they originate from. The risk of rupture grows with increase in size and rupture usually occurs when the aneurysm reaches 5-10mm. Rupture commonly occurs during activities that increase blood pressure and a constant environmental factor that has been associated with increased risk of subarachnoid haemorrhage is cigarette smoking.

Spontaneous subarachnoid heamorrhage (SAH)

Spontaneous subarachnoid heamorrhage (SAH) is a common neurosurgical emergency and accounts for 5% of all strokes. In the UK the incidence of SAH is 10/100,000 population per year. the incidence varies geographically and is about 5 - 15 /100,000 in western European USA, 3.5 in South Africa, and 25 in Japan. In UK, about 5000 to 6000 cases are admitted each year and in USA about 28000. The sex ratio is M : F is 1 : 1.5 and the common age of presentation is 40 - 60 years.

The common causes of spontaneous SAH are:

1. Abnormalities in intracranial blood vessels
    Aneurysms   70 -75%
    Arterio venous malformations (AVMs) 5%
    Moya Moya disease, seen mostly in Japan
2. Abnormalities in blood with bleeding tendency
    Haemophilias
    Other coagulopathies
    Anticoagulant treatment (Eg. warfarin)
    Antiplatelet treatment (Eg. aspirin)
3. Generalized diseases predisposing to haemorrhage
    Hypertension
    Vasculitis
    Collagen disorders such as lupus
4. Intracranial tumours

Spontaneous SAH from ruptured aneurysms is the commonest. Among those with ruptured aneurysms, 15% die before admission to hospital, after admission to hospital, if untreated, 15%, die within the first 24 hours, 15% within 1 day to 2 weeks, 15% from 2 weeks to 2 months and 15% from 2 months to 2 years and about 10% per year thereafter. Even after treatment, the mortality is still high and 6% die from re-bleeding and 7% from vasospasm. 1% of those who survive re-bleeding and 7% of those who survive vasospasm are left severely disabled.
The majority of aneurysms occur around the circle of Willis and 90% are in relation to the anterior circulation while 10% are in the posterior circulation.

Pathophysiology
Aneurysms form due to a weakness of the vessel wall usually at a point of branching where there is a defect in the media of the vessel wall. The tendency to form aneurysms may be hereditary and sometimes there is also a familial incidence. The bulging vessel wall distends to a sac which eventually ruptures. Sometimes the sac can be enormous and result in pres-

sure on adjacent neural structures such as the optic chiasm or nerve or other cranial nerves such as the third or sixth. At the point of rupture of an aneurysm, the rush of arterial blood into the intracranial cavity causes a sudden increase of ICP to nearly systolic blood pressure. This could cause immediate damage to surrounding brain tissue as well as a massive autonomic disturbance that could result in a cardiac arrest. However, the majority of patients survive this episode and get admitted to hospital. The blood in the subarachnoid space causes meningeal irritation leading to photophobia and neck stiffness. Sometimes there could be concomitant haemorrhage into the brain parenchyma causing an intra-cerebral haematoma (ICH) that could result in focal brain damage as well as raised ICP if the ICH is sufficiently large.

Following the initial haemorrhage, very often the point of rupture of the aneurysm is sealed with a thrombus. The presence of blood in the CSF activates a chemical reaction due to degradation of the blood resulting in build up of fibrinolytic enzymes in the CSF. This build up reaches a peak around the 7th to 14th day and is responsible for lysis of the thrombus that had earlier sealed the point of rupture. This results in re-bleeding and on this occasion thrombus formation is impaired due to the fibrinolytic activity in the CSF and very often re-bleeding proves to be fatal.

The presence of degraded blood products in the CSF also contributes to accumulation of chemicals responsible for vasospasm and this results in varying degrees of spasm of main arteries that will eventually cause ischaemia and infarction of brain tissue.

The blood pigment in CSF also damages the arachnoid granulations resulting in poor CSF absorption leading to a communicating hydrocephalus. Hydrocephalus could also be caused by obstruction to CSF flow from intra-ventricular blood clots.

The complications of aneurysmal rupture are

Intracranial
1. Damage to neural tissue at point of haemorrahge due to sudden rise of ICP
2. Focal brain damage from intracerebral haemorrhage (ICH)
3. Raised ICP from ICH
4. Re-bleeding
5. Vasospasm and cerebral ischaemia and infarction
6. Hydrocephalus
5. Epilepsy

Extra cranial (mainly due to autonomic dysfunction)
1. Cardiac arrhythmias
2. Myocardial infarction
3. Pulmonary oedema
4. Gastric haemorrhage
5. Hypo or hypertension

Patients with spontaneous SAH present with sudden onset of very severe headache. The onset is so sudden that patients often recall what exactly they were doing when they were struck down by the headache. Often the headache is accompanied by nausea and vomiting and they may lose consciousness. Due to the presence of blood in the subarachnoid space, they have signs of meningeal irritation such as photophobia, neck stiffness and a positive

Kernig's sign. Sometimes, they also develop a focal neurological deficit with the onset of the headache.

Depending on the extent of brain damage the clinical picture of the patient on admission could vary in severity and has been classified to different clinical grades. The World Federation of Neurological Surgeons (WFNS) suggested the following grades which also seem to correlate with outcome. The WFNS grade which is now used widely is based on the GCS score and is as follows:

WFNS Grade	GCS score	Motor deficit
I	15	None
II	14 - 13	none
III	14 - 13	present
IV	12 - 7	present or absent
V	6 - 3	present or absent

Patients admitted with the above history should have an immediate CT scan which of ten shows the blood in the subarachnoid space and the basal cisterns. In cases where there is a good history but negative CT scan, lumbar puncture and spectroscopy is invaluable. Following SAH, the red blood cells that entered the CSF undergo lysis and it takes several hours for the liberated oxyhaemoglobin to be converted via deoxyhaemoglobin to bilirubin. The enzyme, haem-oxygenase, which is responsible for the process is only found in the CNS. If a period of 12 hours is allowed following a suspected SAH, CSF obtained with a lumbar puncture can be spun down and spectroscopy performed on it. The presence of bilirubin is diagnostic for SAH. This is a very sensitive test for the first 14 days following SAH. The test should be delayed for 12 hours to allow the break down process into bilirubin to be completed, if not, a traumatic tap will be too early to pick up bilirubin and may contaminate the CSF sufficiently to make future test unreliable. The presence of high systemic levels of bilirubin and high levels of CNS protein may give false positive results but there are formulae to compensate for this. Those patients in poor clinical grades are first resuscitated and their cardiovascular state restored with medical means. Angiography is deferred until they improve to a better grade. If there is an immediate threat to life by raised ICP due to an ICH, this has to be removed as an emergency.

Specific effects of SAH

The medical management of SAH is extremely important and is based on the prevention of rebleeding and symptomatic vasospasm. The greatest risk of rebleeding is on the first day (4.1%) and the cumulative risk in the first two weeks is 19%. Rebleeding is associated with a 78% mortality rate and strict bed rest, restriction of visitors, quiet surroundings, adequate analgesia, stool softeners and antihypertensive agents when the mean arterial pressure (MAP) exceeds 130 mm Hg are measures used to try to prevent this catastrophe. Intravenous beta-blockers are popular for blood pressure control since they have a relatively short half-life, can be titrated easily and do not increase ICP. Seizures occur in as many as 25% of patients following SAH (most common in middle cerebral artery aneurysms) and increase the risk of rebleeding. Two anticonvulsants that allow for rapid IV loading, Phenytoin and Phenobarbital, are both used for prophylaxis. Patients in a poor grade and with increased ICP should be intubated and ventilated and care taken to keep the pCO_2 between 30-35 mm Hg (4-4.6 kPa), avoiding excessive hyperventilation which may cause vasospasm and brain ischaemia/infarction. The cerebral perfusion pressure (CPP) should be kept above 60-70 mm Hg.

Vasospasm
Vasospasm mostly occurs 4-14 days after the haemorrhage and is present in up to 70% of patients. Clinically symptomatic vasospasm is present in up to 30% of patients, may lead to cerebral ischaemia and infarction, and is more common in females, young patients, those who smoke, patients who presents in a poor clinical grade and those with large volumes of blood in the subarachnoid space. Patients present with a new onset decrease in consciousness or focal neurological deficit. Conventional angiography is the gold standard for diagnosing vasospasm but the diagnosis can be made reliably as a bedside test with transcranial Doppler. Other imaging modalities including single photon emission computed tomography (SPECT) and perfusion imaging (Xenon CT, dynamic perfusion CT and MRI), have been used successfully.

Prophylaxis for vasospasm:
Prophylaxis with Nimodipine is now standard practice and it improves overall outcome within 3 months of aneurysmal SAH. It appears that Nimodipine may have a neuroprotective effect by blocking calcium influx into damaged brain cells. Current practice is to maintain normovolemia to slight hypervolemia to prevent hypoperfusion. Results suggest that subarachnoid blood removal with intracisternal injections of recombinant tissue plasminogen activator (rTPA) during surgery for aneurysm clipping may carry some benefit.
Treatment for proven vasospasm:
Hypertensive, hypervolemic, and haemodilution therapy (HHH therapy, triple H), the standard of treatment for proven vasospasm, should be reserved for patients with secured aneurysms to reduce the risk of rebleeding.
Hypervolemia - The central venous pressure (CVP) should be maintained at 10-12 mm Hg. The pulmonary artery wedge pressure (PAWP) should be maintained at 19-20 mm Hg.
Haemodilution - The hematocrit should be maintained at 30-35% with dilution or packed cell transfusion to optimise blood viscosity and oxygen delivery.
Hypertensive therapy - Inotropic support and vasopressors may be needed to keep the mean arterial pressure (MAP) between 90 and 110 mm Hg.
Cerebral angiography with transluminal balloon angioplasty has been reported to lead to improved neurologic outcome in 70% of patients with symptomatic vasospasm. It is effective in treatment of large proximal vessels and is not effective in treatment of smaller distal vessels. Cerebral angiography with intra-arterial injection of Papaverine and nimodipine is also effective. Approximately 15-20% of patients with symptomatic vasospasm will have a poor outcome despite maximal therapy.

Definitive treatment of the aneurysm
Both surgical clipping and endovascular obliteration are highly successful treatments modalities. The international subarachnoid aneurysm trial (ISAT) which included mostly patients with small anterior circulation aneurysms showed a 22.5% relative and 6.9% absolute risk reduction at one year in the disability outcome of patients who were treated with coiling compared to those treated with surgery. There are many caveats to the interpretation of this study and the results cannot be extrapolated to all aneurysms. It has however fixed endovascular management firmly in the mind of physicians and the lay public alike. The main concern of endovascular treatment is the paucity of data on the longevity of this form of treatment. The following are broad guidelines:

Indications for surgical clipping include
Presence of a large parenchymal haematoma that requires evacuation
Young, fit patients with a good clinical grade (WFNS or Hunt and Hess grades 1-3)
Giant aneurysms
Complicated vascular anatomy with arteries originating from the aneurysmal dome
Wide-necked aneurysms (the coils escape from the aneurysm and block distal vessels)
Recurrent aneurysm after endovascular treatment with coil embolisation
Patient's wishes

Indications for endovascular treatment include
Patients who are medically unfit for a long general anaesthetic
Patients presenting with a poor clinical grade
Aneurysms located in the cavernous sinus and basilar tip aneurysm
Patients with symptomatic vasospasm who may benefit from endovascular treatment of their vasospasm
Multiple aneurysms not located close together anatomically
Patient's wishes

Timing of intervention
Early surgery within the first 3 days allows for the prevention of rebleeding, the removal of blood clots that may reduce vasospasm and for the use of maximal HHH therapy since transluminal pressure fluctuations are negated by clipping. However surgery is technically more difficult due to brain swelling and fragility of the aneurysm dome with increased surgical morbidity. Delayed surgery removes most of the technical difficulties except for very late surgery that brings the complication of adhesions. However, the aneurysm remains unprotected for this period and rebleeding carries a high mortality rate. It has been found that patients with good grades (grade 1 and 2) fare better with early treatment. This is less conclusive for grade 3 patients and grade 4 and 5 patients should be managed on a case per case basis. Patients with significant hydrocephalus may sometimes improve significantly on their clinical grading with the simple act of placing an external ventricular drain (EVD). Many centres employ endovascular treatment as a first line of management for patients in a poor clinical grade and some centres are using endovascular treatment as the mainstay of treatment.

Management of ruptured AVMs
Ruptured AVMs frequently cause intra-cerebral heamorrhage with or without SAH. The incidence of complications such as re-bleeding and vasospasm are less than that for aneurysm. The aim of treatment is to prevent re-bleeding and if possible excise or thrombose the AVM. This can be achieved surgically where the AVM is in an accessible non eloquent area of the brain. Other forms of treatment are endovascular embolisaton and radiosurgery where gamma rays or X-rays from a linear accelerator are focused to the AVM after stereotactic localization resulting in slow thrombosis of the nidus. This is especially useful with AVMs in surgically inaccessible areas and where endovascular treatment carries a high risk of extension of thrombosis and infarction of eloquent areas of the brain.

abbreviated mental test score 11, 13
abscess 85, 86, 87, 88, 91, 92
acceleration–deceleration 37
acetazolamide 76, 77
Acyclovir 89
ambient 33
ambient cistern 33
aneurysm 96, 97, 98, 100, 101
aneurysms 65, 95, 96, 97, 99, 100, 101
annulus fibrosus 69, 72
anterior vertebral line 48, 49
apoptosis 63, 64
aqueduct 29
aqueduct of Sylvius 29
Arachnoid cyst 57
arachnoid cysts 65
Arteriovenous malformations 95
astrocytoma 65
Astrocytomas 63, 65
atlanto – occipital dissociation 48
Atlanto-axial subluxation 69
atlanto-dens interval 48, 49
AVM 95, 96, 101

Babinski 24
Bacterial meningitis 85, 86
basal cisterns 32, 33, 35, 39, 40, 42
BAX 64
Benign intracranial hypertension 75, 77
BIH 77
bilirubin 40
bitemporal hemianopia 14
Bony tumours 54
brain abscess 85, 86, 87, 88
Brain oedema 27
brain tumours 29, 43, 63, 64

Brown-Séquard syndrome 7

C

cartilage producing tumours 54
cauda equina 53, 54, 59
cauda equina syndrome 71, 72
Cavernous angiomas 95, 96
central neurocytomas 65
Cerebral aneurysms 95, 96
CEREBRAL INFARCTION 81, 82
cerebral oedema 37
Cerebritis 85, 86, 87, 88
cervical spondylosis 52
Cervical stenosis 73
Cervicogenic headaches 61, 62
Chiari 2 75
Chiari malformations 75
chondrosarcomas 65
chordomas 65
choroid plexus tumours 64, 65
Cluster headaches 61
Coagulase-negative Staphylococci 87
Colloid cyst 35, 37
comatose patient 24
communicating hydrocephalus 35, 36
consensual light reflex 17
conus 56
coronal suture 34
CPA 64, 65
craniopharyngiomas 63, 65
Creutzfeld-Jacob disease 89
Cryptococcus 88
Cryptococcus meningitis 88
CSF 27, 28, 29, 32, 33, 36, 37, 40
CT 27, 28, 29, 33, 34, 35, 36, 37, 38, 39, 40, 41, 42, 43
Cysticercosis 90
Cytomegalo virus 89
Cytomegalovirus 89

D

Dandy-Walker cyst 76
DBI 37
Demyelination 28, 29
deoxyhaemoglobin 40
dermatomes 24, 25
Dermoid cyst 57
dermoid cysts 65
Dermoid tumours 27
dermoids 65
Diamox 76, 77
Diffuse Brain Injury 37, 39, 40
disc herniation 69, 70, 71, 72
disc prolapse 49, 53, 54, 72
Discitis 57, 59, 85, 92
dorsum sellae 38

E

E granulosus 90
Echinococcosis 90
Echinococcus granulosus 90
echo time 28
Edinger Westphal 16, 17
Edinger Westphal nucleus 16
Ehlers-Danlos syndrome 96
empyema 85, 86, 91, 92
Ependymoma 56, 57, 65
Ependymomas 63, 64, 65
Epidermoid cyst 57
epidermoid cysts 65
epidermoids 65
Epidural abscess 85, 86, 91, 92
Epstein-Barr virus 89
Escherichia Coli 76
Eschericia Coli 87
esthesioneuroblastomas 64
Extrapyramidal system 20, 21

F

falx 32, 33, 36
falx cerebri 36
FLAIR 28
fluid attenuation inversion recovery 28
Folstein's Mini Mental Status Examination 12
fourth ventricle 29, 33, 35, 36
frontal lobe 38, 39
Fundoscopy 14, 15, 20

G

Gait 22, 23
GCS 24, 26
germ cell tumours 65
GFAP 64
Glasgow Coma Scale 7, 24
Glial fibrillary acidic protein 64
Glial tumours 27
glioblastomas 63
gliomas 64, 65
glossopharyngeal nerve 19
gradient echo 28
Group A Streptococci 87
Group B Streptococci 87

H

Haemophilus Influenza 76, 86
Haemophilus Influenzae 87
HAEMORRHAGE 81, 82
hemiparesis 7
Herpes Simplex virus 89
HIV 89
homonomous hemianopia 14
Horner's syndrome 17
Hounsfield 28, 41
Human immunodeficiency virus infection 88
hydrocephalus 29, 35, 36, 37, 75, 76, 77

hydromyelia 24
hydrostatic pressure 36

I

ICH 81, 82
idiopathic intracranial hypertension 75, 77
intervertebral disc 6, 47, 48, 50, 53, 54, 57
intra cerebral haemorrhage 81
intracerebral haematoma 15
Intracerebral haemorrhage 39
inversion recovery 28
isodense 27, 42

K

Ki-67 64

L

lambdoid 34
lateral geniculate body 14, 16
lateral rectus 15
lateral ventricle 32, 36, 37
lateral ventricles 29, 32, 35, 37
ligamentum flavum 52, 53
light touch 24
Listeria Monocytogenes 87
lymphomas 63, 64
Lymphoproliferative tumours 54

M

Magnetic Resonance Imaging 28
Marcus Gunn 17
Marfan syndrome 96
Marshall classification 39
medulloblastoma 65
medulloblastomas 63, 64, 65
mega cisterna magna 76
meningiomas 63, 64, 65

Meningitis 85, 86, 88, 89, 90, 91
Metastatic 29
Metastatic tumours 54
MIB-1 64
Migraine 61
mini mental state examination 11
MRC Scale 21
MRI 28, 29, 33, 34
Multiple myeloma 54
mycobacterium tuberculosis 57
Myelopathy 69, 71, 72, 73, 74
Myxopapillary ependymoma 56

N

Neisseria Meningitidis 87
neo-vascularity 43
Neural foramina 47, 50
Neurenteric cyst 57
neurofibromatosis 96
neurofilament 64
Neurological examination 10, 11
Neuron specific enolase 64
non-communicating 35
Normal pressure hydrocephalus 75, 77
NPH 77
nucleus pulposus 69, 70

O

Obstructive hydrocephalus 35, 37, 76, 77
odontoid peg 48
oligodendrogliomas 63
oncogenes 63, 64
optic chiasm 16
optic nerve 11, 14, 16, 17
Osteomyelitis 59, 85, 86, 91, 92

P

p21 64

p53 63, 64
Pain sensation 24
papilloedema 7, 15, 17
paragangliomas 65
Paramagnetic 28
parasympathetic 16
Parinaud's syndrome 65
pedicle 50
Perineural cyst 57
pineal cysts 65
pineal parenchymal tumours 65
pituitary adenomas 65
PML 88
Porencephalic cyst 76
posterior vertebral line 48, 49
prepontine 33
Prion disease 89
Proprioception 20, 21, 23, 24
Proton density 28
pseudo tumour cerebri 75, 77
17p 63, 64
pulse sequences 28
Pupillary constriction 16, 17
Pupillary light reflex 16
pyramidal system 20

Q

quadrigeminal 33
quadrigeminal cistern 33

R

radiculopathy 71, 74
Rathke's cleft cysts 65
REFERRAL 5, 6
repetition time 28
Rheumatoid Arthritis 69
Rinne's 19
Romberg 23

S

SAH 95, 97, 98, 99, 100, 101
schwannomas 65
sensory level 7
sensory system 24
septum pellucidum 36
short tau inversion recovery 28
sinusitis 61, 62
Skull fractures 37
Snellen chart 11
Solitary plasmacytoma 54
spinal accessory nerve 19
Spinal canal stenosis 69, 73, 74
spinal cord 47, 48, 52
Spinal stenosis 53
Spinal tumours 47, 54
spinolaminar line 48, 49
spondylolisthesis 69, 73
Spondylolysis 69, 73
Spontaneous subarachnoid haemorrhage 95
Staphylococcus Aureus 78, 85, 86, 87, 91, 92
Staphylococcus Epidermidis 78
STIR 28
Streptococcus Pneumonia 86
Streptococcus Pneumoniae 87
subarachnoid 27, 33, 35, 39
Subarachnoid haemorrhage 39, 61, 95, 96, 97
subdural 37, 38, 40, 41, 42
Subdural empyema 85, 86
subdural haematoma 38, 40, 41, 42
subdural haemorrhage 37, 40
subependymal giant cell astrocytomas 65
subependymomas 65
superior oblique 15, 16
synaptophysin 64
Synovial cyst 57, 58
syringomyelia 24

T

T solium 90
Taenia solium 90
Tarlov cyst 57
temporal bone 36, 38, 41
temporal horn 36
Tension headaches 61
third ventricle 29, 33, 35, 36, 37
Tissue intensities 29
Toxoplasma gondii 89
transient ischaemic attack 5
trigone 32, 36
Tuberculosis 57, 85, 90, 92
Tumour suppressor genes 63

U

uncus 41
upper quadrant hemianopia 14
upper quadrantanopia 14

V

vagus 19
Varicella Zoster virus 89
Vasospasm 97, 98, 99, 100, 101
Venous angiomas 95, 96
Ventriculitis 85, 86, 88
Vestibular schwannoma 33
Visual acuity 11, 14
Visual confrontation testing 14, 15
Visual field 11, 14, 15, 19
Visual fields 11, 14, 15

W

Weber 19, 20
WHO classification 63

www.ingramcontent.com/pod-product-compliance
Ingram Content Group UK Ltd.
Pitfield, Milton Keynes, MK11 3LW, UK
UKHW021321180426
11947UKWH00015B/1366